What others say

"Many women have found that once they quit dairy, their menstrual cycle was more regular and they had less pain and menstrual symptoms."

Rochelle Windust, Naturopath, Australia

"If you're looking for one single food group to eliminate from your diet for the sake of your health, I recommend starting with dairy products. Many of my clients have experienced dramatic recoveries from acne, dermatitis, asthma, sinus congestion, arthritis, migraines and chronic constipation, just to name a few conditions. Milk really is liquid meat.

There's no biological requirement for humans to consume bovine baby food!"

Robyn Chuter, Naturopath, Sydney, Australia

"With 16 years as a holistic skin expert I can strongly agree that becoming dairy free has a positive impact on the skin and gut. Strengthening the skins' integrity as well as reducing puffiness and breakouts or unexplained rash-like appearances on the skin. Thanks to Kris and this book the transition is finally easy and delicious. With joy and passion Kris cuts through the confusion and overwhelm and fast-tracks you back onto your path of inner (and outer) beauty."

Carly Petkovic, Owner of Skin by Carly, Australia

"I have watched Kris over the past years creating the I Quit Dairy online program and writing this book. With this work she opens up her treasure chest and provides you with everything you need to know to start your dairy-free transformation. She is an amazing wizard in the kitchen and the recipes she shares in this book are mouth-watering, easy and super quick. Yet there is so much more to it than cooking. The depth of information Kris shares with you via this book will allow you to ease into this new way of living. If you are looking for an authentic, passionate and down to earth guide to make this transition fun and delicious – you found it!"

Malindi Lovegrove, Founder of The Chocolate Yogi, Australia

"I am a researcher of Leadership and Self Awareness who has worked with more than 3 million people in over twelve countries. Spiritual and physical health are my key resources which enable me to help my customers transform their lives and businesses in the most effective way. When my naturopath told me about the benefits of dairy-free living and that 70% of the world's population suffers from side effects in some way after consuming dairy, I decided to give it a try myself. Today, I can tell you that going dairy-free has transformed my life. After only 2 weeks, I felt better and experienced unknown levels of energy. The most amazing thing is that my improved health boosts my business as well. I need less sleep and think clearer which makes me even more effective in helping my customers fuel their business growth. I can only recommend going dairy-free so you can experience the benefits yourself. It will not only change your health, it will TRANSFORM your whole life."

Jeffrey Slayter, Best-selling Author, International Speaker & Entrepreneur, Australia

"With my knowledge from today, if there was one thing that I could change in the upbringing of my children, it would be to not give them any dairy-products. Yet, if I had done that, then this book would not have been written… For me personally, I can only say going dairy-free has changed my entire life, even though 5 years ago I would not have been able to imagine a life without cheese. Today I always get excited when Kris shares one of her creations with us."

Silke Knuetter, Kris' Mum, Germany

"Kris is so generous with her information, recipes, tips and tricks, and her energy and passion for dairy-free living is infectious. I am a very health-conscious person myself. And even though I went dairy-free before I read this book, I still got so much out of it. My favourite parts are the pantry reboot, the swap guide and the recipe frameworks. Learning from Kris' own experiences and her years of research was incredibly valuable to me. The fact that Kris has been practising a dairy-free lifestyle for many years here makes this guide genuine and practicable."

Miranda C., Wellness Warrior, Australia

First published in 2019 by Food of Tomorrow Pty. Ltd.

© 2019 Kris Goetz

COLLABORATIONS

Are you a health profession who loves the program and would like to support your clients during their transformation while benefitting from our incredible affiliate program? Please contact healthpro@iquitdairy.com.

Are you an outstanding dairy-free food creator, brand or influencer who is looking for collaboration partners with a highly targeted audience? Please contact team@iquitdairy.com.

COPYWRITE

ISBN: 9780648546603

Design & Recipes by Kris Goetz

Cover photos by Kenny Singh (www.kennygphotography.com.au)

Photo on page 144 by Derek Bogart (www.derekbogart.com)

Photos by Anni Ave: Buttermylk, Nozarella, 2 Ingredient Cooking Cream

Photos by Kris Goetz: Power Porridge, Superpower Breakfast Smoothie, Ultimate Banana Yogurt, Power Granola, Pumpkin Pancake, Filling Real Fruit Yogurt, Superpower Seed Bread (gluten-free), Best Peanut Butter, Sour Cream, Walnut Pesto, Green Machine, Green Salted Caramel, Green Mango Lassi, Rich Chocolate Smoothie

Photo by Brenda Godinez (via www.unsplash.com): Açai Bowl

Photos by Amy Pearson (www.amypearsonphoto.com): all other food photos

Editing by Susan McLachlan (www.susanmclachlan.com)

MEASURMENTS GUIDE

Kris uses a 250ml cup and a 15ml tablespoon which equals 3 teaspoons.

OVEN GUIDE

Kris typically uses the oven on fan-force. All temperatures are provided in degrees Celsius. Please note that baking times can vary depending on your oven.

SUBJECTS

Dairy-free diet | Dairy – Health aspects | Dairy-free diet recipes | Weight loss | Low fat diet

DISCLAIMER

The content of this book is for general instruction only. Each person's physical, emotional and spiritual condition is unique. The instruction in this book is based on Kris' own research and experience, and not intended to replace or interrupt the reader's relationship with a physician or other professional. Please consult your doctor for matters pertaining to your specific health and dietary requirements before making any changes.

Find out more about our *I Quit Dairy* online Program at www.iquitdairy.com

To that little voice in your mind,
aka your gut feeling / intuition

May you always have the courage to follow that voice.

This little voice told me for years that I should go dairy-free, yet I didn't feel supported and was unsure if it was a safe thing to do. So I ignored it until one day it screamed at me. When I finally listened I was presented with a completely new world of food: vibrant, energising and delicious. Today I call this the 2nd milk universe.

I hope this book gives you the confidence to follow your inner voice. We are here with you every step of the way.

Enjoy.

I Quit Dairy

The fastest & easiest way to go dairy-free
+ 60 quick & yum recipes

Kris Goetz

Message from Kris

Let's get to know each other. Please go to: <u>www.iquitdairy.com/welcome</u> where I left you a little welcome video.

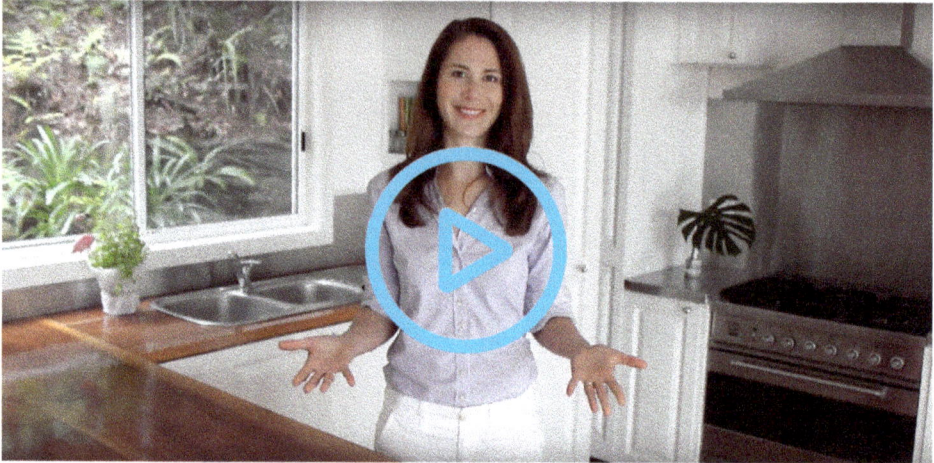

Welcome to I Quit Dairy.

Before we kick off your dairy-free transformation, let me share my motivation and inspiration for creating this program with you.

Back in 2008, I was diagnosed with lactose intolerance and a thyroid disease, which later turned out to be the autoimmune disease Hashimoto's thyroiditis. While my intuition told me that it was time to fully eliminate dairy from my diet, my dietitian told me that instead of cutting out dairy, I actually had to increase my dairy consumption and focus on lactose-free products and cheeses, as they were comparably low in lactose. After a second health professional agreed with this recommendation, I followed their advice. I trusted them, even though I still had this inner voice which kept telling me,

"Kris, your body cannot really deal with this food and it hurts. Why do you continue to eat it?"

At the time, I didn't know any better. It was only in 2014, when I was suffering from a major hip injury and unable to walk, that I discovered the truth about dairy. All treatments didn't work and I was desperately looking for a solution, when my doctor mentioned that inflammation in my body was preventing a speedy recovery. So I did more research into diet and learnt that dairy is highly inflammatory, that science is linking it to more and more diseases, and that it was not only okay but actually really good to live dairy-free. I asked myself,

"Why didn't anyone tell me this before?"

So I cut out dairy completely overnight and within days felt so much more energised. My skin cleared up and my hip finally started to heal. Best of all, I fell in love with food again. After years of calorie counting, I finally felt free. I was able to maintain my ideal body weight despite introducing nuts into my diet and not being able to exercise. I was blown away, not only by the benefits I experienced in my own body, but also by the broader environmental and ethical impact that my diet change had on the world around me. At one point, I thought,

"I want to shout it from the rooftops – everybody needs to know this! This is life-changing."

There I was, deep diving into research, reading every book, checking every super-market for the latest dairy-free products and cooking up a storm creating quick and easy dairy replacements. After all, dairy myths were busted, and my dairy-free lifestyle felt easy and delicious. Today I live the life of my dreams. I am healthy and free from medication and pain. In order to help others and share what I've learnt along the way,

I created *I Quit Dairy*.

This book is what I would have loved back in 2008 when I was first diagnosed with lactose intolerance. *I Quit Dairy* provides the confidence and tools needed to go dairy-free in the easiest, most joyful and delicious way, without overwhelm, or countless hours of research and years of recipe testing. In this book you will receive:

- Answers to the 40 most commonly asked questions, including nutrition, pantry reboot, shopping, cost and time saving hacks, and handling of social situations

- 60 easy and delicious recipes (pssst: they're also gluten and sugar-free) that will help you to turn your current favourite recipes into dairy-free versions

- 20 cheat sheets, checklists and frameworks that will support you in your day-to-day life

I Quit Dairy is your transformation buddy. It's here to help you expedite your journey into an easy, yum and quick dairy-free life. Enjoy the ride.

PS: If you are looking for more support, simply join our Facebook group (search: Dairy-free Heroes) or join the full 8-week I Quit Dairy program at www.iquitdairy.com.

Contents

GETTING STARTED 1

    How this book is structured... 1

    How do I get the most out of this program?....................... 2

    What positive changes can I expect?................................... 3

    Are there any temporary side effects?................................. 4

PANTRY REBOOT 6

    What ingredients can I add to my pantry? 6

    Which foods are traditionally dairy-free?.......................... 8

    Which foods contain dairy? 8

    Food swaps: How can I replace dairy products?............... 10

    Which mylk is best for… ? 12

DAIRY-FREE BASICS 14

    What does lactose intolerance mean? 14

    Why is being lactose intolerant actually normal? 14

    Why did we start drinking milk in the first place? 15

    Do I have to go 100% dairy-free? 16

    Cold turkey or step-by-step? 17

NUTRITION.. 18

    Why consult a health professional? 18

    Why isn't milk the best source of calcium? 18

    Where do I get my calcium? 19

    Kris' favourite dairy replacement all-stars 20

    Quick and easy meal inspirations................................... 20

SHOPPING.. 22

    How to read food labels 22

    Kris' favourite products and brands................................. 23

Cost saving hacks...24
Time-saving hacks 26

FOOD MARKETING..28
Why do I need to know about food marketing?.....................28
Which strategies does the dairy industry use?.....................28
What are common tactics of the dairy industry? 30
How do I know what's right or wrong? 31

GOING OUT 33
How to get your friends on board 33
How to handle work functions 34
What to cook for friends...36
Where to dine out? 38
How to travel on a dairy-free diet? 39

STAYING DAIRY-FREE...41
Why living dairy-free is actually easy? 41
What are the ethical implications? 41
What are the impacts on our environment? 42
How to become more confident? 44
Where can I get more information? 45

GRADUATION 48
Woohoo! Congratulations..48

RECIPES...50
Mylks...52
Breakfast...65
Cheeses...82
Spreads & Dips...98
Pasta Sauces 112
Sweet Treats 123
Nice Cream & Smoothies...129

CHEAT SHEETS 134
RECIPE FRAMEWORKS...144
THANK YOU..148
ABOUT THE AUTHOR 149

GETTING STARTED

How this book is structured

I Quit Dairy is the fastest and easiest way to go dairy-free. In this book you will learn everything you need to know to kickstart your new dairy-free lifestyle. It takes away the overwhelm and guides you through the bite-sized modules at your individual pace. The content is delivered via short and sharp chapters answering the 40 most commonly asked questions, 20 practical cheat sheets and 60 yummy recipes.

Chapter 1: PANTRY REBOOT

You will be introduced to new amazing ingredients that are crucial in a dairy-free pantry; you will know which products you can keep and which products you no longer need. Plus in the Swap Guide you will learn how to replace your old dairy-containing favourites with dairy-free alternatives.

Chapter 2: BASICS OF DAIRY-FREE LIFESTYLE

You will learn what the benefits of dairy-free living are, why dairy isn't the best source of calcium and why being lactose intolerant is actually normal.

Chapter 3: NUTRITION

You will learn how to live dairy-free while maintaining a nutrient rich diet.

Chapter 4: SHOPPING

You will be equipped with a list of our favourite dairy-free products and know how to read labels.

Chapter 5: MARKETING

You will understand why we believe that dairy is normal, natural and necessary, why it is not and how to make your own conscious food choices.

Chapter 6: GOING OUT

You will learn how to handle social gatherings and work functions as well as how to be an awesome guest and host dinner parties.

Chapter 7: STAYING ON TRACK

You will learn about the extended benefits of a dairy-free life that will make it a lot easier to stay dairy-free.

At the end of the book you will be empowered to live a quick, yummy and nourishing dairy-free lifestyle without the feeling of missing out.

How do I get the most out of this program?

YOU will only get out what you put in. That means you have to WANT to make this change.

Mindset. This is the key. Be open and excited about the transition that you are about to go through. It's a journey, so take your time and learn step by step. It's not about binge learning, so don't think that you have to read the whole book in one day. That would actually overwhelm you. Take it easy and trust the process; one topic per week is more than enough. One chapter a day, a new recipe every day—step by step—and your dairy-free life will become a step closer each day. Because every step counts.

Repetition. Read the short chapters multiple times—not just once—because every time you read them, you might get another nugget of information.

Support and community. Go through this transformation with a friend because it's just so much more fun to experiment and try out new things together. You can share recipes, bounce ideas off one another and chat about the emotional part of the journey. Don't just do it by yourself in isolation.

Replacements. Ultimately, it's about finding the replacements that work **for you**. This book is not about cutting out dairy. It is about showing you what replacements are out there, so that once you've found your delicious go-to replacements, you can go with them and just enjoy it.

Expedite your transition. If you would like to expedite your dairy-free transition even further then please be invited to join our I Quit Dairy online program. In the online program you will be supported via:

- 8-week meal plan with shopping list for the whole family so you save time
- Weekly Q&A call where all your questions will be answered
- 40 short and sharp videos so you can learn while you're on the go
- Online Facebook community with the latest products, recipes and much more

Simply go to *www.iquitdairy.com* and join the online program.

What positive changes can I expect?

Some of the positive changes that you might experience along your dairy-free journey:

- **MORE ENERGY.** This is one of the most significant changes for me since I replaced dairy with alternatives. Before going dairy-free, I usually slept between 8 and 10 hours per night and didn't feel energetic throughout the day. After I cut out dairy, I started waking up after only six hours of sleep. My body no longer had to fight the food I was eating and instead was joyfully receiving all the amazing nutrients and energy it needed from the new foods.

- **CLEARER SKIN.** Before going dairy-free, I got to the point with my skin that I didn't go out without putting makeup on first. Within one or two months of cutting out dairy, my skin cleared up so much that today I rarely wear makeup.

- **HAPPY GUT.** Less cramps, bloating, and embarrassing gas. You know what I'm talking about. When your body is trying to digest the fermenting lactose in your stomach, you look like you're in the fourth month of pregnancy. That's just not fun and it's really embarrassing.

- **WEIGHT LOSS.** Especially if your diet is high in cheese. Cheese is super high in fat and salt, plus it is lacking in fibre. Once you replace cheese with delicious and healthy alternatives, the kilos will simply melt away. Be excited about this one.

- **REDUCTION IN THE SYMPTOMS OF COMMON DISEASES**. Science is now showing strong links between dairy consumption and diseases like hay fever, asthma and diabetes. However, make sure that you have a health professional on your side so they can monitor your success and amend your medication and diet according to your personal needs.

- **HORMONAL BALANCE**. From my conversations with health professionals, I also learnt that many women have found that once they quit dairy, their menstrual cycle was more regular and they had less pain and pre-menstrual symptoms. Which is awesome.

- **EMPOWERMENT**. Lastly, this program will open up the door to a completely new world of foods. I always call it my second mylk universe because that's really how it feels. It's empowering to know that we can all take control of our own health and happiness with simple and yummy changes.

I hope that at the end of this program, you feel the same. So, let us empower you! If you have and amazing story to share, please let us know. Send us an email—we'd love to hear from you feedback@iquitdairy.com!

Note: Please be aware that everybody is different and results vary from person to person.

Are there any temporary side effects?

Could there be any negative side effects from going dairy-free? – I'm sorry, yes, potentially.

I was quite lucky and didn't experience any negative side effects. However, if you do, you should know that they are normal and typically only temporary.

Let's start by looking at why we may experience these side effects when we do something good. It's because our body needs to cleanse itself. It needs to get rid of the nasties to make room for the good stuff. It's like when you fall and have an open wound. You need to clean the wound—and that is often painful—and once it's clean, your body can start healing.

So, let's have a look at headaches. This is not necessarily only because you have cut out dairy, maybe it is because you're also moving towards a healthier diet in general: less processed foods, less sugar, less pesticides, less nasties. It means your body is going through a cleansing process. Stay calm and take it easy; give your body time to rest and be gentle. From my own experience, I know that headaches are really no fun, allow your body to cleanse and go through this process—it will be getting better very soon. Also make sure you get enough water. Adding more water can help a lot to support your body to get rid of nasties, plus it keeps you hydrated.

Besides cleansing headaches, withdrawal symptoms can be another side-effect. Withdrawal? Yes, let's have a look at cheese. Cheese actually contains addictive compounds, which is why some people can get mild withdrawal symptoms when they stop eating dairy cheese—especially pizza. According to a study performed by the University of Michigan, pizza is actually the most addictive food there is. Yes, even more addictive than Coke or chocolate. This is due to the combination of fat and salt, and the high concentration of casein (a protein which is in dairy). As we digest it, casein turns into a morphine-like compound that induces feelings of happiness.

Just think about it for a second. Do you remember that super happy face that babies have when they have just finished breast feeding? They even look a bit drunk. Nature is incredible, so it designed mother's milk to be slightly addictive to make sure that babies continue drinking it. Dairy, which is the mother's milk of a cow, is no different. Hence, you might experience withdrawal symptoms. Hang in there, drink plenty of water. Stay calm. It's gonna be all right, very soon.

You might also have FOMO (fear of missing out) because all your friends are having pizza with tons of cheese and you can't. Seriously. Hang in there. Things are getting better. We will show you super handy and delicious replacements that will make it easy for you to say no. Be prepared. Your friends might soon want to try all your incredible foods as well. Lean back and wait.

We highly recommend you work with a health professional to make sure that you are ready to go and that you get the most out of your transition. If you are looking for a new health professional, someone who supports you and is aware of the benefits of a dairy-free lifestyle, and you are not sure where to go, please reach out. We have a long list of amazing health professionals and are happy to help you. Simply email healthpro@iquitdairy.com. We're looking forward to hearing from you.

PANTRY REBOOT

What ingredients can I add to my pantry?

To start, let's have a look at your pantry and give it a nice refresh.

The first thing we'd like to do is to introduce you to all the **newbies**. Here at *I Quit Dairy*, we believe that instead of quitting something, it's all about adding in the good stuff and finding replacements that work for you. We focus on new ways of eating and don't fight the old. So, let's get your pantry really full with lots of new, amazing foods.

Here are nine go-to, dairy-free ingredients.

1. **Nutritional yeast**. These are tiny, wholesome flakes, and there are a couple of brands that produce them. You can get them at health food stores, or particularly online. They are really, really good for creating a cheese flavour in whatever meals you create.

2. **Tahini**. It's ground sesame butter that you can buy unhulled or hulled. It's amazing for hummus and other dips, so try it out. You can even get it at Coles and Woolies.

3. **Coconut cream**. The reason why I always buy coconut cream instead of coconut milk is that they are usually priced exactly the same, with the only difference being that coconut milk has more water, which you can simply add yourself. It's pretty much a third to half a cup of water that I add to one cup of coconut cream if a recipe asks for coconut milk. Coconut cream in general is amazing for cooking, so give it a go.

4. **Nuts**. Yes, I'm all about the nuts.

    a. **Cashews**. Our go-to nuts for cheeses, cooking cream—everything that's really smooth—they also make an amazing mylk that doesn't even split, so a good one to remember.

b. **Almonds**. Maybe the most universal ingredient of all. You can even turn almond butter into our delicious traveller's mylk while you're on the road. They are so good.

c. **Macadamia nuts**. They give you a really, really rich and fatty mylk which is just to die for, especially in desserts.

5. **Arrowroot flour**. It's a thickener, which is really useful, especially if you make your own cheeses like a soft cheddar or our Nozzarella. It's a white powder. All health food stores stock it, and you can also have a look in Coles and Woolies to see if you can buy it there.

6. **Turmeric**. Turmeric is a spice that is really good at combatting inflammation. My secret tip: Adding a little bit of pepper boosts its effect tenfold. Plus, it gives cheese this really lovely yellowish colour, so keep an eye out for this one.

7. **Cacao powder**. Yeah, not cocoa powder. Look for cacao powder, that's the dry part of the cacao bean, nothing added, simply ground up. You can add it to your smoothies or homemade chocolates. Yes, it's a must-have.

8. **Cacao butter**. The oil from the cacao bean. You can get it in different forms, usually either as little buttons or some companies sell it as a whole block. Just see what you feel more confident working with and check the prices as well. Usually you find it close to the baking section or in the health food section, also in health food stores or online.

9. **Nut mylk sieve**. This is something you really should invest in, and it's not that expensive (you can find organic cotton ones in our shop online at *www.iquitdairy.com/shop*). Alternatively, you can simply use muslin or a really thin tea towel. Straining your own mylks gives them an amazing texture. Once your mylk is blended up, you simply pour everything through the sieve, et voilà, you have beautiful, smooth mylk.

So, I hope this has inspired you to get creative and start playing around with new ingredients.

What are your favourite ingredients? Are there any ingredients you had no clue existed before you started your dairy-free journey? Let us know!

See appendix for your cheat sheet.

Which foods are traditionally dairy-free?

This is the second part of our pantry refresh. This time, we check which foods you used to eat before and can keep. We call them the **keepers**. We divided the keepers into five categories.

1. **Whole foods**. They are the save choice and naturally dairy-free—everything that doesn't have a label, like fruit and vegetables for example, and many more. Real foods that don't have a label, they are our number one staple.

   Note: Foods in categories two to five are often dairy-free, however it's not guaranteed. Take a look at the labels of the various alternatives that are available and identify your favourite dairy-free brands. Watch out for those that do include any form of dairy.

2. **Condiments**. Your hummus, your guacamole, your mustard, your Worcestershire sauce, your favourite tomato sauce, even your chilli sauce and your barbecue sauce—foods like this.

3. **Dressings**. A traditional Italian or French vinaigrette.

4. **Snacks**. You can keep your falafel, your chips, the unflavoured corn chips, as well as the traditional potato chips. Also don't forget your rice cakes, wedges, popcorn and olives.

5. **Sweets**. We all love our sweets. I promise not all of your sweets need to go. You can keep your raw cakes and your bliss balls, as well as your dark chocolate, not to mention your jams and sorbets. Most of the time they are fine. Delicious, ripe fruit is always really, really great as well.

What were your favourite surprises? The foods you thought had to go, and now you realise you can actually keep them. Share it with our Facebook Community (Dairy-free Heroes), so others can learn from you.

See appendix for your cheat sheet.

Which foods contain dairy?

The third and last part of our pantry refresh: Which foods are better left out of your pantry?

We divided this group into four categories.

1. **The obvious ones**. Milk, cheese, yogurt, cream, butter, milk chocolate. All of these foods contain dairy.

2. **On second thoughts**. When you think about it a little more, you'll likely realise that dairy is also a main ingredient in the following foods:

   a. Baked goods: especially pastry, which traditionally contains butter as a key ingredient.

   b. Condiments: many bread spreads contain dairy, like Nutella.

   c. Dips: most low-fat dips (manufacturers often use yogurt to reduce the fat content), tzatziki obviously. In fact, most store-bought dips contain some form of dairy.

   d. Pasta sauces: everything that's creamy, as well as pesto.

   e. Creamed soups.

   f. Dressings: like ranch or American dressing.

   g. Savoury snacks: flavoured chips, check the label, especially for milk powder.

   h. Sweet snacks: muesli bars often contain yogurt or milk chocolate.

   i. Fried foods: when you are eating out, check whether the chef is cooking with butter or oil.

   j. Whey protein powder: whey is a by-product of cheese production.

   k. Smoothies: they sometimes contain yogurt, milk or whey protein powder.

3. **The not so obvious foods**. These are the ones you might not think would contain milk.

   a. Processed foods: like cold cuts or pre-cooked dinners.

   b. Potato fries: sometimes there is milk powder in them.

   c. Dark chocolate: a couple of brands like Cadbury as well as the 78% dark chocolate from Lindt still contain milk.

     d.   Some coconut products: sometimes they are just coconut-flavoured dairy products.

4. **The hidden ones**. You might not expect these products to contain dairy at all.

     a.   Soy chai lattes: I love my soy chai lattes, unfortunately most powders contain milk powder.

     b.   Medication: some pills have a lactose coating.

     c.   Flavourings.

     d.   Wine: Some wineries use milk protein in their fining process.

     e.   Probiotics: always go for the vegan option.

See appendix for your cheat sheet.

Food swaps: How can I replace dairy products?

Let's talk about swapping, so you know how to replace your old dairy foods with new exciting dairy-free foods.

- **Milk**. You can replace a dairy milk with soy mylk, almond mylk, or with any other mylk; like coconut or seed mylk. There is an endless list of dairy-free mylks now. In the US you even get pea mylk because it is higher in protein. Start trying different mylks and soon you'll find your favourite.

- **Yogurt**. So many people love their yogurt. How can you replace it? There are coconut yogurts out there as well as coconut kefir, and also soy yogurt and almond yogurt. If you're keen to experiment, you can also try replacing yogurt with silken tofu. When it comes to your desserts and topping your fruits with yogurt, you can also be a bit more creative and make your own puddings with chia seeds, tapioca, or sago pearls.

- **Cheese.** The availability of nut or soy-based cheezes in grocery stores is rapidly growing, plus of course you can make your own cheezes. If you want to keep it easy you can simply replace cheese with veggies, like a thick slice of eggplant on pizza or avocado on chilli. Nutritional yeast is another great replacement, especially for parmesan in recipes like risottos or pesto. For my favourite super quick lasagne cheeze, mix some water with 2 tablespoons cashew butter, juice of ¼ to ½ a lemon, 1 tablespoon nutritional yeast and season with salt. That's it – easy, refreshing and delicious.

- **Whipped cream**. Instead of using the traditional whipped cream, you can use avocado or coconut based whipped cream, which you can make yourself. There are even store-bought rice-based creams. Keep an eye out. They are even available in spray cans.

- **Cooking cream**. A lot of people ask me, "How are you replacing cooking cream?" My favourite replacement is actually a mix of 50% cashew nuts and 50% water, quickly blended. Just add both to the blender and blitz them; it's really quick. You can always have it handy and it's also cheaper than normal cooking creams. Another alternative is silken tofu or some nut butters. If you have a creamy sauce and you want to add a little bit more texture, you can simply add some almond butter. Lastly, a flour-water mix also works pretty well, especially for gravy sauces.

- **Butter.** Are you wondering what you can smear on your bread? One option is avocado. You can also try tahini or a nut butter. For cooking, you can use a high-quality olive or macadamia oil. Most of the time, I use water and it works perfectly fine. Some people use coconut oil, so just try and find the right replacement that works for you.

- **Chocolates**. We have a wide range of vegan chocolates available nowadays. They are all dairy-free and available in many different flavours from mylk to strawberry to salted caramel. Pretty much everything is out there. You can of course also go for your traditional dark chocolates. Typically, the higher the cacao content, the more likely it is that your chocolate is dairy-free.

- **Ice cream**. I'm really getting excited about this one. You can make your own ice cream from frozen bananas and coconut cream. That's basically all you need. If you are out and about and you just want to have a scoop of ice cream, grab a scoop of sorbet instead.

BONUS: Check out *www.iquitdairy.com/bookbonus* and watch our short 5 minute video on food swaps.

I hope these replacement ideas have inspired you to just test and try what works well for you. Happy swapping and enjoy your new and exciting foods.

    See appendix for your cheat sheet.

Which mylk is best for... ?

This list is your starting point for picking the right mylk for your needs. Learn more about the different mylks out there and then you can choose which mylk you want for what.

1. **Soy mylk.** The most famous dairy milk alternative, which has been used especially in Asia for hundreds of years. In recipes you can replace it one on one, just be mindful of the difference in taste, as soy mylk is less sweet than dairy milk. Also when you buy soy mylk, please make sure you get a soy mylk that uses the whole bean not just soy protein isolates.

2. **Almond mylk.** This is the second most common mylk out there at the moment. Whether you make it yourself or not, it's amazing for cereals—you don't even have to strain it. Just leave the fibre in and enjoy it as it is. Almond mylk is a true all-rounder. Little word of warning: Do not put it in your coffee, it'll separate and doesn't look nice. The ones used in cafés usually contain thickeners and sugar, so always double-check. When you buy almond mylk in-store ideally watch out for at least 7% almond content as some only have 2%—No, I am not kidding.

3. **Cashew mylk.** Another really good one because it doesn't separate when you add it to hot coffee or tea. It's creamy and smooth. Unfortunately, cashew mylk is rare to find in stores, but super easy to DIY.

4. **Macadamia mylk.** Macadamia is very rich and creamy. It's perfect for rich desserts or something heavier.

5. **Rice mylk.** Is a little bit sweeter and really light, making it the perfect match for pancakes or baking. It's my mum's go-to coffee mylk.

6. **Oat mylk.** Is also good for baking. It's nice and creamy. Please note, if you cannot tolerate gluten, your body might not like it. I can't have oat mylk, for example.

7. **Sunflower seed mylk**. This sounds a bit awkward, doesn't it? I try it in our live Dairy-Free Kickstarter events and it's always a big surprise. It tastes really good. Just add some dates to it for a really nice and distinct flavour. It is the perfect mylk for anybody who wants to or has to go dairy-free, and also has a nut allergy.

8. **Hemp seed mylk**. Hemp is now finally considered an official food in Australia, after it had already been available in the US and Europe for a long time. And no, it has nothing to do with smoking! Hemp seed mylk has a nutty flavour and is high in protein, so it's the perfect match for your post-workout smoothies.

9. **Coconut mylk**. Another rich mylk that has a lot of its own flavour. It works perfectly in curries or rich and delicious desserts.

I hope this mylk guide has given you a bit of guidance and some ideas to try different mylks for different purposes. Let me know what your favourite mylk is. We'd love to hear from you.

DAIRY-FREE BASICS

What does lactose intolerance mean?

Let's talk about lactose intolerance, and what it actually means.

From birth, we all produce an enzyme that is called lactase. Lactase helps our digestive system to break down the lactose that is present in our mother's breast milk. Lactose is also called milk sugar as it breaks down into glucose and galactose, which are absorbed into the bloodstream and provide necessary energy.

Usually at the age of five, the production of the enzyme lactase ceases naturally, as we no longer depend on our mother's breast milk past this age. It's how our bodies are designed. It is totally normal. There is nothing abnormal about it.

If people who no longer produce the enzyme lactase continue to consume dairy products, the lactose in milk ends up in their gut, unprocessed, where it starts to ferment. The normal side effects of this are bloating, gas, diarrhoea, plus damage to the gut flora.

Why is being lactose intolerant actually normal?

One fact to set the scene:

- At least 70% of the global human population is lactose intolerant.

- The other 30% are so called 'lactose persistent'. Their bodies continue to produce the enzyme lactase past the age of five.

Based on these numbers, I ask you to re-think what is 'normal' and what is not.

Here at *I Quit Dairy*, we believe that being lactose intolerant is actually normal and that you should not feel bad about it. It's actually the way nature designed us, because after the age of five we can digest proper food and are no longer dependent on our mother's milk, and therefore don't need the ability to digest lactose any longer.

Feel normal and good about being lactose intolerant.

Why did we start drinking milk in the first place?

In order to understand why some people are lactose persistent (those who continue to produce the enzyme lactase past the age of five), we need to understand the history of why we started consuming dairy in the first place.

7,500 years ago some people started consuming dairy, especially in European and Arabic areas. When they had a really, really bad harvest they still needed to be able to eat and survive. Instead of killing and eating their livestock, which would have meant a relatively early ending to their food supply, they started to think, "Hmm, we can drink our mother's milk, so why wouldn't we be able to drink some of the cow's milk in order to survive?" So that's what they did.

Apparently just consuming the dairy straight from the cow resulted in diarrhoea and often death. Later, people found out they could process and ferment the milk, and thereby create cheese, yogurt and butter, which they were able to tolerate better. This was a good way for them to get a lot of nutrients and survive. Over the centuries, the genetics of these people changed and their bodies continued to produce lactase post-childhood. This genetic change (called lactose persistence) is estimated to apply to only about 30% of the global population. The rates of lactose intolerance in South America, Africa and Asia is considered to be closer to 100%. So, I guess what's normal and what's not depends on your perspective.

Now, let's go back to the 1920's. That was pretty much where the big push for milk really started. In that time, four key things happened:

1. High infant mortality.

2. The first milk pasteurisation machine was invented.

3. Some people (e.g. factory owners) wanted to encourage others (e.g. their staff) to stop drinking alcohol.

4. There was an increase in research following the realisation of the potential of using food to benefit health. Milk was considered the perfect food at that stage because it was high in carbohydrates, high in fat and high in protein.

As a result, people believed milk was a good food to nourish us all. Back then, health professionals and the government started to push dairy into our diet.

Then the next big push came after World War II. Milk powder was a main source of nutrition for the infantry and soldiers. After the war ended, the industry was left in a state of over-production and needed to come up with new ways of selling their product. Also, the government provided its support for the industry as many people's jobs depended on the continued production and consumption of dairy products. One of the results was that 'school milk' and similar concepts started because it was still believed that milk was a very healthy food.

I hope this little excursion into our history helps you to understand where this all came from.

Do I have to go 100% dairy-free?

Some people ask me, "Do you have to live 100% dairy-free in order to get the benefits from a dairy-free diet?" This really depends on your personal 'why'. If you are allergic to dairy or you have an autoimmune disease and dairy is a key trigger for that, then it's highly recommended that you go 100% dairy-free.

On the other hand, if you are doing it for other reasons, a step-by-step process might be a good idea. You could start with replacing one dairy product category entirely, like milks or dips, and start to explore and experiment with new foods. For example, if you want to have a coffee with milk, from now on you could have your coffee with hazelnut, almond or soy mylk. This small change will alter the taste without adding any sugary syrups. Go for it—get excited!

I don't believe that we have to do everything 100%. Take that pressure off and just start to tune in. As always, listen to your body.

What about you? Are you 100% dairy-free or not?

Which kinds of foods are you struggling with to replace?

Which foods are the ones you don't want to give up for whatever reason?

Cold turkey or step-by-step?

So, what's the best way to transition into a dairy-free life? Basically, there are two options.

1. **Cold turkey**. This means you change from one day to the next, or to be more precise, start your 100% dairy-free journey NOW.

2. **Step-by-step**. In this case, you either swap

   a. food category for food category

      Start with a new mylk for your cereals. Next, replace the cheese in your sandwich with a dairy-free dip. Then use the DIY cooking cream, and finally try a nut cheeze or your favourite dairy-free mylk for your coffee.

   b. meal type by meal type

      Start with a dairy-free breakfast, move onto dairy-free lunch and ultimately transition to your dinners.

I'd love to share my experience.

When going both dairy-free and gluten-free, I went **cold turkey** once I found out that it might actually help me from a health perspective. I re-tested it two or three months later by temporarily adding dairy and gluten back into my diet, and I immediately suffered from the same symptoms I had experienced before. I knew why I went 100% dairy-free and going cold turkey forced me to find alternatives.

When I adopted a plant-based diet, I used a **step-by-step** approach, and I'm really glad I did this. I started with just my breakfast and did that for a full week. The next step was looking into my lunch options. Then I added a couple of vegan dinners and quickly transitioned towards 100% five days a week. I was really loving my food, and then I felt confident to go all-in for a full month, pretty much cold turkey for a month. It took me about three months before I wanted to give it a go. Now, I don't look back and the final cold turkey phase was pretty easy for me as I already had some go-to favourites and the basics were set.

It's really up to you. Trust your gut and try out what you feel comfortable with.

NUTRITION

Why consult a health professional?

Why do I recommend you have a health professional, like a dietitian, a naturopath, or a nutritionist on your side? It's not because this is a scary thing to do or anything like that. It's about having someone on your side who can give you the confidence that you're on the right path, and also show you the benefits of going dairy-free, which is really powerful. For me, it was crucial to have a health professional on my side because I have an autoimmune disease. When I first started, I wasn't aware of this and only saw a health professional when I started having palpitations. Ultimately, I was able to reduce my medication throughout my journey. Especially if you have something like an underlying disease, make sure you have a health professional on your side.

Be really critical about who you choose because they need to be your partner. Make sure they agree with your values and share the same vision for your health. There are a lot of dietitians and nutritionists out there who believe going dairy-free is actually a good thing. If you are looking for a health professional in your area, there are multiple ways to find one. First, you can search online or ask your friends, and you can also drop us a line. We might be able to find someone who's the perfect match for you. It's always good to bounce off a health pro.

Why isn't milk the best source of calcium?

"Wow—but Mrs. Smith always said to drink your milk because you need to get your calcium."

Let me bust this myth wide open: milk is simply not the best source of calcium.

1. When we compare milk and the calcium content by cup with other foods, it's right up there. When we look at it from a calorie perspective, it's actually near the bottom. Trust me when I say there are a lot of better alternatives.

2. When you have a look at the countries with the highest consumption of dairy, they are usually also the ones with the highest rates of osteoporosis. Just think about it.

3. In 1976 Harvard University initiated one of the largest investigations into chronic diseases in women called the *Nurses Health Study*. Two of the surprising findings were: 1. They could not find a link between milk consumption and fracture risk; 2. They also found that calcium supplements did not provide protection against hip or other bone fractures.

    Furthermore, when we think about our bone-health, many dairy alternatives in contrast to dairy also offer a wide range of nutrients such as magnesium, potassium, boron and vitamin K which holistically support your bone-health.

4. Milk doesn't contain any fibre, which is a key ingredient in all our natural foods, and helps our bodies to digest them better. The other sources of calcium, which we will introduce you to later, are all also rich in fibre.

5. Lastly, there are many other things in milk that might not really be good for us. Does it make sense that we have to drink or consume cow's milk in order to get the nutrients we need? Dairy is the mother's milk of another species—essentially, it's the growth formula for a calf to grow from 50kg to 200kg in less than one year. Just think about all the hormones.

Do you still think milk is the best source of calcium?

Where do I get my calcium?

Let's have a look at alternative sources of calcium. The following four foods are actually really good sources of calcium and do not contain any dairy at all.

1. **Leafy greens**. Yum, delicious salads. (especially kale, bok choy and broccoli, while—from a purely calcium perspective—spinach, chard and silverbeet for example have a high-oxalate content which hinders our absorption of calcium).

2. **Soy beans**. In form of tofu, tempeh or edamame beans. If you make a stir fry or a curry, add some tofu or tempeh next time.

3. **Tahini**. This Arabic sesame seed paste is so delicious, especially in hummus, or you can make salad dressings with it (simply combine tahini, lemon juice and some water).

4. **Almonds**. The dairy-free all-rounder. The ideal snack. Always a good choice.

To finish off, let me give you one last **digestion hack** so you get even more out of your calcium sources. Always combine your calcium sources, especially the leafy greens, with a source of **vitamin C**. Next time you make a salad, add some capsicum or put lemon in the dressing and your body absorbs even more of this vital mineral.

See appendix for your cheat sheet.

Kris' favourite dairy replacement all-stars

This chapter is all about motivating you to explore and find your favourite dairy re-placements. To make this easier, here are my five go-to dairy alternatives.

1. **Nice cream**. You can make your own ice cream and it's freaking easy and super delicious. Check out our recipe.

2. **Self-made dips**. Like hummus and beetroot dips, for example. Oh my gosh, they are so amazing, tasty and delicious—and are done in pretty much three minutes.

3. **Green smoothies**. Yum! Full of calcium, delicious nutrients, and so refreshing. And a little kitchen hack: if you add a little bit of cacao powder, you can't even see the greens.

4. **Cashews**. Cashews are another absolute all-rounder. You can make your own cheese, mylk and don't forget about our two-ingredient cooking cream!

5. **Tahini**. I didn't really use tahini often before I changed my diet. Today I spread a thin layer of it on bread, use it in our dips as well as in our salad dressings.

Quick and easy meal inspirations

Let's look at some meal inspirations. What can you eat if dairy is off the plate?

At first, this might seem hard because dairy is in pretty much every dish.

1. **Breakfast**

    a. Make your own cereals or muesli with a mylk.

    b. Green smoothies. They are super yummy and unbelievably quick to make.

    c. Lastly, your fruit and açai bowls—who doesn't love these?

2. **Lunch**

    a. Wrap or sandwich. Just replace the butter and cheese with a yummy dip.

    b. Salads. Always a good and healthy option.

    c. Leftovers. If you have anything left over from dinner—like a curry, stir fry or chilli—just add a big portion of salad to it and you're good to go.

3. **Dinner**

    There's seriously nothing to miss out on. You can still have:

    a. Burgers. Indulge in creamy sauces, like guacamole or our beetroot-almond dip.

    b. Barbecue. Use dairy-free dips & salad dressings.

    c. Pasta and pizza. Just be creative with what you put on top of it and try out a few different things until you find your go-to recipes.

4. **Snacks**

    a. Vegetables with dips.

    b. Nuts & fruit.

    c. Olives.

    d. Falafel with hummus.

    e. Sweet potatoes. In Japan, they sell sweet potatoes as street food. So good! They're really easy take-away food—put them in your bag and snack on the go.

Over to you. What are your favourite dairy-free foods to eat throughout the day? Share a photo or recipe on social media and tag us #iqd, so others can be inspired.

See appendix for your cheat sheet.

SHOPPING

How to read food labels

We want you to be very confident in picking dairy-free products. Dairy has a million different names on the ingredient labels. It starts with milk, yogurt, butter, and can also be less obvious, such as casein and whey.

But there is a shortcut.

When you look into the allergy section right at the bottom of the ingredients list, it states, "Contains: …", and if milk is listed, stay away from it. Some products have, "May contain: …" or "May contain traces of: …" If the product *may* contain milk, whether you choose to buy it really depends on 'why' you decide to live dairy-free. If you're allergic, seriously stay away from it. The reason why milk is listed under "May contain traces: …" is cross-contamination.

So, what does cross-contamination mean?

Let's look at a chocolate factory that produces both dairy chocolate as well as dairy-free chocolate on the same product line. In this case, there is the risk that leftover dairy is still present in the so-called dairy-free product as it may not have been cleaned properly. This is called cross-contamination.

Also look for **buzzwords** like, *dairy-free*, *vegan* as well as *paleo*. However, just because these labels are on the product, it doesn't necessarily mean that these products are actually healthy. Please read the labels and look for ingredients you know. An approach that I take is, if I can cook it myself, it's quite likely on the save side. Stay away from everything that you cannot pronounce and have no clue what its purpose is in your foods. For example when I buy mylks I look for organic, activated nuts with at least 5 or even better 7-10% nuts and no sugar, no thickeners and no oils – these ingredients simply don't need to go into mylk. Stay on the healthy side.

In order to make it even easier for you, we've put together a list which includes different names of milk products. You can find this list at the end of the book, together with all the other cheat sheets and check lists.

Kris' favourite products and brands

In order to help you locate good dairy-free products on your first shopping tour, we have put together a list with my favourite dairy-free products. If you are a visual kinda person, go to *www.iquitdairy.com/bookbonus* for the video version of this chapter.

I tried to reduce the list to five dairy-free favourites. That didn't work out, so here are my 11 favourite dairy-free products.

1. **Bonsoy**. When I go into a coffee shop and have my soy chai latte, I make sure that they have Bonsoy. It is THE best soy mylk you can buy and the ingredients are very clean.

2. **Nudie.** When it comes to yogurt, I really like and enjoy the plain Nudie Coconut Yogurt, and I have to smile when I read the label: "Cows need a holiday too."

3. **Over the Moo**. Let's talk about ice cream: have you heard of Over the Moo yet? They have an ice cream truck driving around Sydney. Yes, there's sugar involved, and I only have a tiny little spoon of this ice cream every now and then… and always remember how easy it is to whip up your own Nice Cream.

4. **Chia Pods**. One product that I really enjoy is Chia Pods. You can get them pretty much everywhere and they're a great way to replace your snack yogurt—just get a little chia pudding. My favourite is the coconut and my hubby loves the chocolate one.

5. **Cashews**. I just couldn't resist adding cashews to my list. Why? Because you can do pretty much everything that you want with cashews, so they are my go-to nut. Be nuts.

I know cheese is a biggie, so I actually have three favourite dairy-free cheeses for you:

6. **Nozzarella.** This cheese is perfect for pizzas and every meal you want to top up with some melting cheese. Only down side - it's a little bit hard to locate.

7. **Peace Love Vegetables.** Ideal for spreading on a piece of bread or sandwich. It is just divine with a bit of dill. Really, give this one a try. It is quite pricey—it's definitely worth it though.

8. **Sprout & Kernel**. This is the star on our cheese platter every Christmas. Yes, even though I live dairy-free, I am responsible for the cheese platter for all my friends. Funnily enough, there are never any left-overs for us to take home… Definitely try their *pepper* cheeze it really is a winner.

It's hard to pick my favourite dairy-free chocolate (for more info on this topic, make sure you read our free Dairy-Free Chocolate Guide).

9. **Chocolate Yogi.** I'm a little bit biased because these guys are actually friends of mine. I really like the Chocolate Yogi and they have heaps of different flavours, so try them out. My fave is *Head in the Clouds*. Oh, and not to forget they do heaps of charity work as well.

10. **Pana Chocolate.** They are Melbourne-based, and pretty much conquer the whole world at the moment, which is so cool. Dairy-free chocolate everywhere, even at the airport.

See appendix for your cheat sheet.

Cost saving hacks

So many people think that eating dairy-free has to be expensive, that's nonsense. So, I've put together my four best money-saving hacks.

1. **Do it yourself.** Mylks, ice cream, cooking creams and nut butters. These four products you really do not have to buy. Just blend them up yourself. It's quick and it's easy.

2. **How you cook**.

    a. **Use water.**
    When you fry, you can use water instead of expensive olive or coconut oil.

b. **Coconut cream**.
If a recipe asks for coconut milk, instead use a mix of coconut cream and water. Coconut milk and coconut cream are usually the same price, with the only difference being added water to the milk.

c. **Use the whole thing.**

- Cauliflower: use the stem in your potato mash.

- Celery: instead of just using the stalk. You can use the leaves for salads or to spice up another dish.

d. **Leftovers**.
Freeze them, so that next time you're about to run to a restaurant because you don't have time to cook, you can just warm up your frozen dish and enjoy.

3. **How you shop**.

a. **Go to your farmers' markets**.
Especially just before they close, that's when the best sales are on.

b. **Join a co-op**.
You usually have to pay a little upfront fee, while the discounts you receive throughout the year usually make it really worth it.

c. **Buy seasonal.**
Everything that's in season is heaps cheaper than out of season produce.

d. **Consider frozen fruit.**
Especially blueberries; they can easily be half price if not even cheaper than fresh ones. Stay away from frozen bananas, because they are usually just a complete rip-off. You can easily do it yourself: get a whole box of bananas, peel them, chuck them in the freezer and you're all set up for your smoothies or nice cream.

e. **Buy in bulk**.
Especially with nuts and seeds. They are not perishable—not easily perishable at least—and you can share them with a couple of friends and save some decent money.

4. This is **the cheeky one**. Have friends who really like inviting you out for dinner, and let them pay for your dinner :)

Do you have any more cost-saving hacks? We'd love to hear from you.

See appendix for your cheat sheet.

Time-saving hacks

In our busy world, *time* is the most precious resource we have. Therefore, I've put together my five time-saving hacks.

1. **Preparation.** Cut down on your cooking time. If you want to have rice for dinner, soak it first in the morning. When you come home and start your cooking, your rice will be done in 10 instead of 20 minutes.

   Also, overnight oats are a good option for breakfast. In the evening when you are relaxing, just mash banana, add some oats, add some water and put it in the fridge. Then in the morning, all you have to do is grab and go.

2. **Get a good food processor**. I'm no Michelin chef, and I bet you're not either. So why not cut your veggies with a food processor? You just chuck them in and, zzzz, they're all done, all the same size, super quick.

3. **15 to 20 minute recipes**. Everybody thinks you need to cook for ages in order to get a great meal. This is nonsense. There are a lot of recipes out there that only take 15 to 20 minutes. Arm yourself with your favourite ones, and get cooking.

4. **Planning ahead**. Make a meal plan so you know what you're having on each day throughout the week. Go shopping once for the whole week. This way you don't have to worry about what you're going to eat in the evening.

5. **Cook in batches**. If you put passion into cooking a dish, why not just make twice as much and freeze one portion. So, next time you have a busy night, you simply take it out of your freezer and enjoy a really easy and delicious meal.

Now over to you. This is all about creativity, and we love to hear from you. What sneaky time-saving hacks do you have? Did your grandma give you an amazing tip that everybody should know about? Send us an email to feedback@iquitdairy.com so we can spread the word.

⊞ See appendix for your cheat sheet.

FOOD MARKETING

Why do I need to know about food marketing?

You might wonder why food marketing is a topic here in the first place, when we are talking about diet and lifestyle. Well, on a daily basis we are bombarded with a million different marketing messages. Sometimes they can be quite subtle and it's hard to see through them; it is important to make your own informed and conscious decisions.

Marketing is my passion and I have years of experience in the field. I even did my Masters in Marketing here in Australia. Now, I would love to share what I've learnt along my journey so you can make better decisions.

You will learn some of the strategies and techniques the dairy industry is using to lure us into consuming more of their products and, ultimately, how you can make your own conscious decisions about what is actually good for you.

Which strategies does the dairy industry use?

Let's talk about the strategies the dairy industry is using. Fundamentally, they want us to believe that milk and other dairy products are:

- **Normal**
- **Natural**
- **Necessary**

The three key strategies that the dairy industry uses:

1. **Availability (normal).** Dairy products are woven into so many other products. They are available everywhere. It starts with school milk and con-

tinues with pizza. You can find dairy in pretty much anything. You can always drizzle some cheese on top of your meal and you can have milk with almost everything. If you have kids, you'll notice that most kids' snacks contain some form of milk, especially muesli bars. It really is everywhere, and because it's everywhere, we think it's **normal**.

2. **Fairy tale world of happy cows (natural).** Happy farm, happy farmers, happy cows. That's what they build into their packaging and also into their marketing messages. They say, "We've done this forever. Cows need to give milk so they are not in pain—they were created to give milk and it is the most **natural** thing." But it's not.

3. **Kids (necessary).** They picked a very, very distinct target audience to be as successful as possible, which was mums with kids between 5 and 12. If you want to learn more about this, check out the Dairy Australia website. So why is this target audience perfect for them? Because mums want to do the best they can for their little kids; they want to see them flourish and grow and give them everything they need. So the mums are told, "You need to include dairy in your child's diet because it is the best source of calcium, and without enough calcium, your kid might get weak bones or even get osteoporosis later in life." Subsequently, mums think they have to give their kids milk because they want them to be happy and healthy. That's their strategy to make you think it's **necessary**.

Later on, we will bust all those myths. For now we'll focus on the marketing.

There is another strategic layer supporting their natural, normal and necessary messages and that's **creating confusion**. There is heaps of research out there that has been around for years, which proves that dairy is neither necessary, natural, or normal. However, in order to keep the myths alive, the dairy industry strategically supports charities and research. This leaves people confused, unsure of what's right or wrong, so makes them continue with what they used to believe. That's how we humans behave; it's our natural reaction to confusion—going back to what we believe is 'normal'. In the following section where we talk about their tactics, we share two links so you can see for yourself how they do it.

What are common tactics of the dairy industry?

Now it's all about their tactics - what they are doing and how they make you think that dairy is normal, natural and necessary.

The first tactic is their advertising.

1. **Fun**. They bring a lot of fun into their ads, which makes us smile. Think about the 'water slide tester' and the claim that dairy is 'legendairy'.

2. **Product placements**. As with many other products, dairy is also often present in movies. Think about 'Eddy the Eagle' where the little one always drinks milk and at the end he participates in the Olympics. More subtle placements are also employed, such as seeing milk on breakfast tables or actors buying milk in the local food store. This makes dairy appear to be part of normal life.

3. **Testimonials**. Especially celebrities who participated in the Milkstache campaign—a campaign that showed celebrities with a milk moustache. By being in these commercials, these celebrities made us believe that because **they're** drinking milk, it's a good thing because they should know what a good diet looks like, shouldn't they?

These three tactics are creating a fun experience; we smile when we look at them. They make us believe that it is good and normal to consume dairy, so we don't want to miss out on it.

4. **Creating confusion or doubt**

    a. **National Asthma Council of Australia.** Follow the link and you will see a post entitled 'Why dairy is not necessarily linked to asthma'. Scroll down to the very bottom and you will see a disclaimer that the information has been provided by the dairy industry.

    b. **Dietitian Association of Australia**. They talk about lactose intolerance and about how you are still able to consume dairy despite your lactose intolerance diagnosis, and even that it is necessary. This is the Dietitian Association of Australia—who else would you believe? Again, when you scroll to the very bottom of this leaflet you see that this information was brought to you by 'Dairy Australia'.

I don't believe it's wrong that companies support research, it makes sense and can actually be a good thing, as long as they publish the results correctly or not at all. Businesses have a responsibility towards their customers too. If there is a chance that someone improves their asthma symptoms by cutting out dairy, we should make sure that they get this information and that sponsoring doesn't stand between patients and their health.

Be really aware of this. Whenever information is being provided to you, scroll down and see who's funding it. I hope this information helps you to open your eyes.

How do I know what's right or wrong?

To help you make your own conscious decisions when looking at marketing and advertising messages, we have created this four-step process:

1. **Do your own research**. This is crucial. You need to find your own arguments and find resources that **you** can trust. Be critical, especially when things are mentioned that sound strange or don't make sense to you. Always do your own research before you accept any information as true. Please go and do your own research– no argument is as strong as the one you discovered yourself. This is what I have done.

   To make it easier for you, we have included a 'further reading' section every day throughout the program. In there, we recommend some films, books and audiobooks, as well as cookbooks. It is a great starting point for you to do your own research.

2. **Be critical**. Don't believe everything you read in the newspaper. I mean, there was an article out there once stating that Diet Coke is better than water after exercise. That's a little bit stupid, so don't always believe what you read. The way I approach it is when I read an article and think "Ah, this is weird" I first think about who could benefit from that kind of research. Then, I try to figure out if there's a financial supporter or someone funding this study. By doing this, you can quite quickly find out where the information is coming from. If you then want to go one step further, you can try to see the raw data and make up your own mind. First of all, don't believe everything you read.

3. **Take your time**. I'm serious about this. Take your time. If you can't find a dairy-free alternative, just keep looking around. Usually there are dairy-free alternatives, be it in a restaurant, be it at a festival. Look around and be creative. You will find a nice dairy-free alternative I'm sure.

4. **Be aware of the power of your own choice**. Just one example. Last year, Sainsbury's sales for vegan cheese exceeded their expectation by 300%. What happened next? Sainsbury's launched their own vegan cheese line. It's a really, really small target audience that has created this change by creating a demand. So when you buy a product, be aware that you are putting your money into it, and by doing so, you give power and energy towards creating this new world that you want to see. By supporting alternative companies and products, you are supporting them and their growth. Be really, really aware of where you put your money and what change in the world you want to see—every single dollar counts.

I promise, it gets easier over time and soon you'll know what's true and what's not. You can differentiate and look through all the marketing messages assertively, and soon enough, you'll become really quick at making your own decisions. It takes a bit of time and practice, so be patient.

GOING OUT

How to get your friends on board

Social gatherings on any special diet can be tricky. If your friends or family invite you, you want to make it as easy as possible for them, so they keep inviting and visiting you.

I have five hacks to help you be a better guest on a dairy-free diet.

1. **Answer all questions seriously**. If your friends or family have questions regarding your dairy-free diet, take the time to answer all of them. Even though it might sound a bit weird to you. For example, if someone asks you, "Quick question. Is coconut milk actually dairy-free?" Don't start laughing, just say, "Yes, it is." Maybe even add that you were surprised as well.

2. **Recommend easy tweaks**. If someone asks, "I've invited you, and I'm not quite sure what I can cook for you," ask them what they plan to cook. For example, if they want to make a salad, check what kind of dressing they're using. If their dressing contains yogurt or any other dairy products just ask them to keep the dressing on the side, and if they have some vinegar or lemon and some olive oil so you can make your own dressing and also enjoy the salad. That's a really easy thing to do. When it comes to sharing plates and different dips, ask them to get some hummus, because hummus has a relatively high likelihood of being dairy-free if it is store-bought. Also tell them what your favourite brands are, so that the host doesn't have to read all the labels.

3. **Be a source of amazing, quick, easy, and yummy recipes**. Especially if your friends want to find out more and really go above and beyond, be there for them. I'm so blessed with my friends and my family as they do go above and beyond. Today we share recipes, they cook some of my recipes and send me

33

new recipes they discover, which I find really, really amazing. Be the source of healthy, yummy, quick and easy recipes, and inspire the people around you.

4. **BYO** (Bring Your Own). I always offer to bring something when I'm invited, especially desserts, because they're really tricky. Usually there's heaps of dairy involved in desserts and if you don't want to end up with a plain fruit salad (don't get me wrong, fruit salads can be freaking amazing), if everybody else is having chocolate cake, bring your own and really WOW everyone at the table with your dairy-free creations.

5. **Be prepared**. It really depends on where you're going; sometimes going out can be a tricky one, especially if there's lots of cheese and cream about. In this case, I recommend you eat beforehand. Seriously. This way you are not starving and you don't feel like you're missing out. Have something really delicious before you leave and then go and be an amazing guest. Just pick at some little dairy-free bits and pieces.

Bottom line … the secret to being social on a special diet is to make it easy for others and not preach. People might be interested in what you're doing, simply wait until they ask you questions.

How to handle work functions

I know work functions can be quite daunting, especially when you have just started changing your diet. You don't want to be that outsider, you want to simply enjoy these work functions as much as you can! These are my five hacks to really enjoy your next work function.

1. **Check in with the organiser**. If there is an event coming up, usually the organisers will ask you for your dietary requirements, so make sure to get back to them. Instead of just sending an email, I always pick up the phone and give them a quick call. I ask if they already have an idea of where we're going and what we'll have. This way you get a clear idea and sometimes together you can work something out that's easier than what you both thought. Again, it's about making it easy for them.

2. **Check in with the venue**. Depending on who is organising the event, it might be easier to check directly with the venue. Tell them, "Look, I don't

want to make a big fuss about my dietary requirements, could you share with me what you're planning to cook? Could you maybe make something dairy-free for me on the side? That would be absolutely fantastic. Thank you so much." This might be a really good shortcut, as some event organisers don't feel comfortable and don't know how easy it can be to work something out that suits everyone.

3. **Propose a venue**. If your team wants to go out and you know there's this amazing place that everybody would love, plus they also have something for you, propose it. Don't go somewhere hard-core where they only have dairy-free foods; suggest somewhere that caters for everybody.

4. **Be prepared**. Bring your own foods. If you know there is a tea time, traditionally the cakes are baked with butter. What I always do in this case is to bring a little cake for myself in my handbag, which I then just pull out and enjoy. It blends in with what everybody else is eating and nobody realises that I brought my own food. The best thing is that I don't have to miss out on anything. Or eat beforehand, and always have some nuts in your bag. If it's a whole day workshop, make sure you have something with you because working on an empty stomach isn't good.

5. **Say you have an allergy**. It's sometimes good to just say you have an allergy even though you might not. Saying you have an allergy makes it seem a lot more serious. I've been to places and simply asked them, "Is that dish vegan—so no dairy or eggs?" and they've said "Yes". Despite the fact that I was actually allergic to eggs, I didn't specify this more clearly. Unfortunately, one day a piece of banana bread contained eggs and I had an instant reaction—it was mild, but still not good. When I told them about it, they said, "Oh, you have an allergy. You should have told us." When they hear the word allergy, alarm bells go off for waiters and they will double and triple check as they don't want to risk anything. So take your time, explain it to the waiter or to whoever you are dealing with, and try to find something that works out for everybody. Informing them that you have an allergy can sometimes be quite helpful.

To finish off, I want to leave you with two more … let's call them thought bubbles.

1. **Be strong**. If you decide to go dairy-free because you want to or even have to do it 100%, I suggest that you stay strong. There are reasons *why* you decided

to go dairy-free. When you're looking at a dessert menu and all the options contain dairy and you think, "Oh, I'd really love to try the mousse au chocolate," remind yourself what it does to you. Go through the process in your head; imagine you're eating it and think what you will get out of it. Is it joy, or pain? You've been there, you've done that. So choose wisely.

2. **See it as an opportunity**. This really excites me. Some colleagues might see you as 'that health freak', while it could also be a door opener. It could help you network and have completely different and exciting conversations. It's really powerful and, I mean, who doesn't want to talk to a healthy person and know more about it? It's okay if this doesn't feel right at the beginning; you might feel a bit unsure of how to respond to critical questions. You will know when the time is right when you can use this opportunity to glow and shine.

What to cook for friends

How can you host amazing, dairy-free dinner parties without your friends feeling like they're missing out? These are my four guidelines:

1. **Portion size**. Just because something is healthy, nobody should go home starving or still be hungry. So, make sure you plate up big portions.

2. **WOW**. Make your dishes **wow**, so when people take a spoonful they just go, "Well, this was incredible, and I can't believe that's actually dairy-free! Wow, this was really, really good!" Make sure your food has this kind of effect on people, so they understand why you're doing it. It's not just because you have to, it's because it's amazing and it's delicious.

3. **"Aha!"** Make your guests think, "Aha, this is dairy-free? I had no clue." We sometimes make a big Mezze plate as a starter where we have some vine leaves, antipasto, falafel and veggies with hummus and beetroot almond dip. People are just dipping and eating, and at one stage probably five or ten minutes in they might wonder, "Is this all dairy-free?" And you say, "Yeah, it is." They might think, "Oh, I could do this myself. It's so easy."

4. **Easy**. The food you serve should be easy to prepare because you want to inspire others to cook foods that you can enjoy as well, just like the Mezze plate.

Don't we all want to inspire others? The way to do this is not by spending hours and hours in the kitchen behind closed doors. It is about making dairy-free options easy and accessible to others. Make sure you follow these rules, and I bet your next dinner party will be just amazing.

To finish off, I pulled together three dinner party ideas.

1. **Summer**

   Starter: A little soup like a gazpacho.

   Main: Barbecue with heaps of veggies, salads and of course your favourite dairy-free dipping sauces.

   Dessert: Chocolate-dipped fruits. Everybody loves these.

2. **Italian Night**

   Starter: Antipasto or bruschetta.

   Main: Pasta with your favourite sauce, like a lovely tomato sauce or a pesto.

   Dessert: Delicious ice cream. *Prepare it in front of your guests so they can see how easy it is.*

3. **Asian Fusion**

   Starter: Rice paper rolls with soy sauce (or tamari as gluten-free alternative) or a yummy satay sauce.

   Main: Curry

   Dessert: Chia pudding with a really delicious mango on top. Pretty much like the sticky rice mango dessert that you find at some Asian places.

As I said, it's all about having yummy and easy food, and remember when you catch up with friends, food shouldn't be the centre of your night. The centre should be the conversations you have. Those flashbacks to your shared memories, telling stories and laughing together. That's what it's all about when you meet friends, so enjoy your next dinner party.

See appendix for your cheat sheet.

Where to dine out?

To help you find restaurants where you can enjoy dairy-free foods, we have pulled together this restaurant guide with the most common types of cuisine.

1. **Vegan and raw food restaurants**. They don't use dairy whatsoever.

2. **Paleo restaurants**. I would say at least 95% of their meals are dairy-free. Just watch out for yogurt, parmesan or butter. The staff at paleo restaurants usually know exactly what you're talking about when you ask for dairy-free options and are happy to help.

3. **Organic and whole food restaurants**. They tend to cook from scratch, so when you ask them if they can make anything dairy-free or if they can recommend anything, they are pretty good in helping you out and making something specifically for you.

4. **Asian restaurants**. In Asia, they traditionally don't use any dairy. It's a relatively save choice. Check out a Chinese or a Malaysian place for example.

5. **Indian restaurants**. With Indian restaurants, you need to know from which part of India the food originates, some parts use a lot of yogurt and ghee. Always check with the staff; they know their food quite well. Curries tend to be made just with coconut cream, so check for that. I love curries from real Indian places, so hot and spicy.

6. **Lebanese restaurants**. Traditionally the Lebanese cuisine is really low in dairy, watch out for yogurt or lebna in some of their dips.

7. **Italian restaurants**. Gosh, I love my Italian pizza. They are so easy to amend; it's usually just about taking off the cheese. Sometimes, you can simply replace cheese with avocado without having to pay extra—check with the waiter. One little heads-up: If you go to an Italian place for the first time, always ask if they use butter in their frying process, even for tomato sauce, and if they could replace it with olive oil for you.

I hope these restaurant tips gave you a good idea and some confidence in going out again.

And this is how I ask for any changes or special meal creations:

1. I usually check the menu online and call the restaurant before I go there and ask if they have anything for me.

2. When I'm there, I put on my biggest smile and I introduce myself to the waiter with, "Sorry. I'm your most painful customer for today, but I'm really nice and super grateful once we've figured out what I can have." That usually makes them smile and prevents any problems.

3. Don't trust in the waiter to know what your requirements are and which dishes you can have. If you want to enjoy your meal take ownership and come up with suggestions.

Honestly, I never have any issues with ordering food, and I'm not just dairy-free. I always order plant-based (vegetarian without eggs or dairy) and gluten-free dishes. Pretty much free, from their perspective, of everything. In the end, the meals usually turn out quite amazing.

Now, I'd love to hear what your favourite restaurants are, so I can check them out as well.

See appendix for your cheat sheet.

How to travel on a dairy-free diet?

I don't know about you, I love to travel and food should not get in the way when I'm out somewhere in the world exploring new places.

This is my two-step process to stress-free and yummy travelling.

Preparation. Seriously, be prepared if you travel with a food allergy or a special dietary requirement.

1. **Online research**. Check out Facebook groups, Trip Advisor, Yelp, and Happy Cow to get an initial idea about your destination as well as recommendations from others about restaurants and other places to eat.

2. If you stay in a **hotel**.

   a. Send them an email and check what options they have.

b. Call a day before you arrive to remind them of your dietary requirements and if they have any milk alternatives for breakfast or if you should bring your own. I always offer to bring my own. Most of the time, this strategy works out and they have soy milk.

3. **Self-contained apartments**. My preferred option, because I have a fridge and can create whatever food I'm after, which makes it a lot easier for me. Everybody is different, so try what feels good for you when it comes to different types of accommodation.

4. **BYO** (Bring Your Own). Breakfast is usually the hardest meal for me, also being gluten-free, which is why I usually bring my own. If you have no issues with gluten, breakfast should be easy for you. I take our Everyday Cereals, plus the Deluxe Traveller's Mylk. That's my on-the-road breakfast plus some local fresh fruits, which most hotels provide anyway—and then you have this deluxe delicious breakfast. Nothing to miss out on.

5. **Inflight meals**. Today, airlines offer countless special meals. Pick your favourite dish. Remember, if you need to change planes or even have a stop-over, you can try a second meal at the airport.

At your destination:

1. Check out **supermarkets.**

2. **Restaurants**. I plan my day tours around the restaurants I really want to visit. If I want to go to a special restaurant, I'll look for tourist attractions in that area and try to combine them.

In 2016, I went to the oldest vegetarian place in Rio de Janeiro and, oh my gosh, this place was just amazing! Then when I went to Buenos Aires—that Italian place—they went above and beyond my expectations and I enjoyed the most delicious pizza ever. In 2017, I've been completely blown away by China, Beijing—I had amazing food there without knowing any Mandarin.

You see, there are all these tiny little places around the world that you can explore. I hope this has motivated you to try the different amazing, healthy foods that are out there.

STAYING DAIRY-FREE

Why living dairy-free is actually easy?

Going dairy-free can be easy, while staying dairy-free can be a very different story. Once you decide that you want to live dairy-free, you need to have some tools in place and know *why* you are doing it. I live gluten-free as well, and staying gluten-free is a lot harder for me than staying dairy-free. This is because the only person who benefits from my gluten-free diet is me. Yeah nice, however sometimes when I get a real artisan home baked bread, I simply cannot resist. So, I might have a little piece and risk bloating and a bit of pain.

Being dairy-free on the other hand is complete liberation for me, and allows me to love my food again. Plus, it's about being able to do more—to have a bigger impact than just on my own body. That's what I want to share with you today. It's all about the ethical benefits as well as the environmental benefits of living dairy-free. At the end, we've wrapped it all up with a couple of awesome hacks which make staying dairy-free a lot easier for you.

What are the ethical implications?

Let's have a look at the ethical impacts of consuming dairy.

I had no clue about this when I started my journey.

I thought it was the most natural thing that a cow gave milk, and even that it actually had to be milked in order to not feel any pain. During my own research, I found out that's actually not true.

The dairy industry is not a pretty industry.

It's not this fairy-tale world that we all envision: a world of cows grazing on a paddock, with calves jumping around and we just take the surplus. In fact, these cows are 'raped'—sorry, that's the official term. They are artificially impregnated every year so that they can continue producing milk because, after all, the milk we are drinking is mother's milk. Milk from a mother cow that is meant to be fed to her calf. That's why cows produce milk. The calf is taken away within the first 48 hours after birth in order for us to have the milk that we like to drink. Instead of sucking on their mum's udders, the mothers and calves are separated. What happens next depends on the farm. Have a look at Dairy Australia. Most calves are kept in individual fenced-off sheds or in small groups of calves, and then a car drives by to feed them with milk. The good thing— they do still get cow's milk. Still, they don't have the closeness to their own mothers, and meanwhile the mothers are back on the production line. Once the calves are big enough, if they are female, they become a dairy cow; if they are male, they will end up as veal meat or potentially kept for breeding.

I urge you to do your own research.

Start with Dairy Australia and see what the best dairy in the world looks like because that's what they show.

Two more things:

1. Due to the use of machines for milking, the cows' udders get infected. That's why the dairy industry and the government have established legal thresholds for pus as well as blood in milk. Not to mention that this causes the cows a great deal of pain.

2. These dairy cows are specifically bred so that their milk production is increased and we can take the most milk from them. In fact, I find it quite strange that we talk about milk 'production'. Due to the increased productivity of the dairy cow, their life expectancy sits between four to five years, instead of their natural lifespan of around 20 years.

So, think about this information and let it sink in. Do your own research. For me, understanding and stopping my support of the dairy industry is a huge reason that makes being and staying dairy-free super easy.

What are the impacts on our environment?

Now that we have covered the ethical impact of the dairy industry, it's time to consider the environmental impact on our world.

Once I started thinking about it, there was one thing that didn't make sense to me. Think about the global population of dairy cows—there are millions if not billions. Cows need to eat as well, which means that we need to feed them. Instead of using that food to feed other human beings who are starving, instead we give it to dairy cows to produce milk. Even more staggering, we have to grow this huge quantity of food somewhere, hence the alarming rates of rainforest deforestation we are witnessing today.

Some interesting facts are:

- **Dioxin**. 93% of all dioxin emission comes from the production of animal products. Not just dairy, also meat. Still, it's 93%. One fact that really put things in perspective for me.

- **GMO**. Most GMO (genetically modified) foods are fed into the animal agriculture industry, with the highest amount going to dairy farms. Some people are concerned about GMO soy and they only think about tofu, whereas in fact, the majority goes straight to the dairy and meat industries. This means that people who consume dairy and meat might be consuming second hand GMO foods. (Note: In Australia we are lucky as we only grow GM versions of canola and cotton)

- **Water.** 1,000 litres of water are required to produce 1 litre of milk. Why? It's because the cow itself needs to drink water, plus the vast quantities of grain they eat needs water as well to grow. That's a massive mismatch and a lot of waste. 1,000 litres of water to produce 1 litre of milk—water that we could otherwise drink ourselves.

- **Waste.** A farm with 2,500 dairy cows produces the same amount of waste as a town of 411,000 people.

Let this information sink in. If you want to know more about it, I would love to recommend the documentary 'Cowspiracy'. Again, educate yourself, do your own research on the environmental impact and get in touch; let us know if you have any questions or comments.

Another good thing about steering away from dairy products and picking a dairy-free sorbet instead of ice cream is that you are making an impact straight away and your own ecological footprint on this earth is immediately reduced.

How to become more confident?

In order to support yourself in staying dairy-free and continuing your journey, we have put together four strategies that can help you.

1. **Community**. As with anything, change is easier in a team. Don't do it by yourself—find your own dairy-free community. Here at *I Quit Dairy*, you are already part of one community, we're so pleased to have you here—reach out and find other communities as well. Have a chat with your friends and family, you might be surprised by some of them already living dairy-free. Also have a look at Facebook groups; maybe there are some in your local area. Search for 'dairy-free', 'milk allergies', 'no casein', 'lactose intolerance' etc. Also, vegan, paleo and raw food groups can be really insightful and helpful too. There are many groups, especially over in the US. The issue with the US-based groups is that some of the products are not available here in Australia. Nevertheless, go for it and give it a try.

    If you are in Australia on the Central Coast, we have the 'Central Coast Vegans', which is a Facebook group that is really supportive and welcoming. Even if you only want to go dairy-free and not vegan, people in this group will share recipes, places to go and answer all sorts of questions. Plus, you'll stay up to date when it comes to new products and get-togethers. Check out different groups and see which ones you like.

2. **Be open-minded**. It's all about experimentation. When you start your journey, remember to try different replacements. Try different mylks. Try nut cheeses. Having a positive mindset is crucial as well. It's not about cutting anything out, it's about exploring and finding your new favourites. For example, you can make a super delicious chocolate mousse out of avocado, banana and cacao. Seriously, this is amazing. There are so many new things to discover.

3. **Research**.
    a. Create your own little repertoire of go-to recipes. Again, 15-20 minute recipes. Try to steer away from recipes that take longer—at least during the week. Make sure you like the recipes and they fit into your lifestyle. This will make staying dairy-free so much easier.

b. Watch documentaries, read books and articles. Learn more about the food we are putting into our bodies. Food Matters TV (fmtv.com) and Netflix have a massive library of really, really inspiring and insightful documentaries with heaps of interviews with health professionals.

c. Look for dairy-free bloggers you like. Who inspires you?

4. **Nutritional education**. Consider doing a nutritional course. I have done this. There are courses that will teach you the basics of nutrition in 40 hours. Plus, you'll get a certification at the end. The certification process forces you to actually learn and digest the basics of nutrition, which helps if friends or colleagues have some questions. Honestly, food is just so important; we should all know more about how it fuels us.

5. **Stay in touch**. Subscribe to our newsletter, we will keep you updated with the latest scientific research and new recipes.

I hope these strategies will help you to stay dairy-free. Because it's not only okay, but actually amazingly good to live dairy-free. Think about it. You can change both your world and the world around you with the food choices you make.

Where can I get more information?

I'm always talking about doing your own research. These are my five favourite films and documentaries, books, and blogs. Use them as a starting point and go from there.

Let's start with the films.

1. **What the Health.** Includes many links and heaps of information on dairy and its health impacts, as well as how food industries influence our decisions (available on Netflix).

2. **Cowspiracy**. All about the environmental impact of our food choices (available on Netflix).

3. **Raw The Documentary**. About a couple in their sixties running around Australia on a completely raw food diet. For 366 days, they ran a marathon each day, raising awareness for alternative medicine, the power of food and animal

cruelty. A couple of years back, she healed her breast cancer and is now thriving more than ever before.

4. **Hungry for Change.** The second film from the creators of Food Matters TV. It reveals the power of food for our health and how industries are influencing us to consistently make the wrong food decisions (available on Netflix & FMTV).

5. **Fat, Sick, and Nearly Dead.** From a Sydney guy who went on a revolutionary journey to just drink juice and thereby heal himself (available on FMTV).

Over to my five favourite books:

1. **The Cheese Trap** by Dr Barnard. In this book, he takes a scientific look at cheese. Backed by research and his own experience, he describes the impact of dairy on our health.

2. **Whole** by Dr Campbell. A holistic view at our food industry and how our current diet is benefiting specific industries, not just the food industry.

3. **Miyoko's Kitchen** (The Homemade Vegan Pantry: The Art of Making Your Own Staples) by Miyoko Schinner. She provides a wide range of amazing dairy-free staples. She is one of my biggest cooking inspirations.

4. **Crazy Sexy Diet** by Kris Carr. An engaging and honest mix of nutritional advice combined with super delicious recipes. Yum!

5. **This Cheese is Nuts** by Julie Piatt, the latest plant-powered cookbook from Rich Roll's wife, dedicated to dairy-free cheese in which she shares all her secret little kitchen hacks. Become your own cheese maker.

How about my five favourite blogs?

1. **Kris Carr** from Woodstock in the US. She calls herself a wellness warrior and cancer thriver. Kris is the main character in the documentary *Crazy Sexy Cancer* and author of the New York bestseller, *Crazy Sexy Diet*.

2. **Oh She Glows** from Canada. Everyday easy and delicious recipes.

3. **Minimalist Vegan** from Canberra. Food for both your tummy and thoughts.

4. **Healthy Eating Joe** from Sydney. Amazing food photos and yummy recipes.

5. **Live, Love, Nourish** from up on the Gold Coast, a nutritionist focused on all things dairy and gluten-free. She is a source for healthy eating and nutritional background information, as well as an absolute kitchen whizz.

Lastly a list of my go-to websites to start my nutritional research:

1. **Nutrition Facts**. Home of the latest science packaged in more than 2,000 fact-based videos. It is a really nice platform to start your nutritional research. (*www.nutritionfacts.org*)

2. **FMTV.** Food Matters TV - the Netflix of health and wellbeing (*www.fmtv.com*)

3. **Food Matters.** The blog and home of recipes that goes hand-in-hand with FMTV. (*www.foodmatters.com*)

4. **Beck Health.** For a quick start into nutritional science, a great self-paced fast-track. Their courses are split into different topics and start with a 40 hour program. I did a course here and really enjoyed their content. Everything is well explained and the exam at the end helps deepen your knowledge and turns bland theory into actionable steps. (*www.beckhealth.com.au*)

5. **Integrative Nutrition** for all things body, mind and soul. Many of today's leading wellness coaches studied here or promote it, including the FMTV team, Kris Carr and Melissa Ambrosini. If I was starting my journey today, I would enrol with them. It is a self-paced online program which takes about one year, depending on your engagement. (*www.integrativenutrition.com*)

GRADUATION

Woohoo! Congratulations

Woohoo! You made it. The first seven days of your dairy-free journey. Well done. So, what have we learnt over the past seven days?

Chapter 1: We started with **refreshing your pantry**. We welcomed in new ingredients, kept quite a few of the old staples, and then said goodbye to some nasty dairy-containing foods. We also went through a swap guide that I hope gave you a good idea of how to replace certain foods.

Chapter 2: We went through the **dairy basics**. We questioned if dairy is normal and why we started to consume dairy in the first place.

Chapter 3: We moved on to **nutrition** and learnt where we get our calcium from. We also learnt that milk is actually *not* the best source of calcium.

Chapter 4: We went **shopping**, had a look at what products are out there and learnt how to easily identify dairy-free products in the supermarket.

Chapter 5: Next up was our **food marketing** day. We looked into the different strategies the dairy industry is using, as well as their tactics, and how you can empower yourself to see through them, and make your own conscious decisions that are good for your body.

Chapter 6: We looked at the **social aspect** of living dairy-free, how to be a good guest and an amazing host; how to easily handle work functions, and finally how to eat out, as well as which restaurants to pick.

Chapter 7: Lastly, it was all about **staying on track**. It's key to understand why dairy-free living is not only good for us and our bodies, and also better from an ethical and environmental perspective as well.

Graduation

I hope you feel well equipped with all of this information and you're ready for the next steps.

Just a little reminder, as mentioned before, do your own research. Find resources you trust. We have a massive list of movies and books for you to start with, and really, I urge you to do your own research as well.

So, what's next?

- Let this book come alive by joining our *I Quit Dairy* online program. The online program also includes:

  8-week meal plan with shopping list for the whole family so you save time

  Weekly Q&A call where all your questions will be answered

  40 short and sharp videos so you can learn while you're on the go

  Online Facebook community with the latest products, recipes and more

- Please share your feedback with us! We'd love to hear from you and learn from your experiences. If you have any questions, comments or would like to share your own journey with us, please send us an email to feedback@iquitdairy.com.

- If you enjoyed this book and know someone who could benefit from a dairy-free lifestyle as well, please feel free to share the love.

RECIPES

MYLKS

How to Strain Mylk 52

Cashew Mylk 53

Almond Mylk...................................54

Sunflower Seed Mylk........................55

Coconut Cream 56

Love Mylk.......................................57

Vanilla Brazil Mylk..........................58

Deluxe Traveller's Mylk 59

Buttermylk......................................60

Pistachio Date Mylk.........................61

Macadamia Orange Mylk.................62

Chocolate Hazelmylk.......................63

BREAKFAST

Everyday Cereals 64

Power Porridge 66

Chia Pudding with Apple Sauce 68

Chocolate Overnight Oats...............69

Peach Melba Overnight Oats...........70

Superpower Breakfast Smoothie 72

Açai Bowl.......................................73

Ultimate Banana Yogurt 74

Power Granola.................................75

Pumpkin Pancake............................77

Smooth Coco Chai Quinoa.............79

Filling Real Fruit Yogurt..................81

CHEESES

Parmesan...82

Crumbly Macadamia Cheeze............83

Herbed Cheeze Wheel.....................84

Melting Pizza Cheeze 86

Soft Cheddar...................................87

Nozzarella 89

Cheezy Nacho Sauce 91

Ultimate dairy-free Queso
with Chili & Nachos........................93

Golden Sweet Potato
Pumpkin Pizza 95

Pear & Walnut Salad with
Crumbly Macadamia Cheeze............97

SPREADS & DIPS

Quick German Spelt Bread 98

Superpower Seed Bread 100

Cashew Cream Cheese 102

Newtella.......................................103

Best Peanut Butter.........................105

Hot Spread...................................106

Tomato Spread 107

Hummus.......................................108

Guacamole 109

Beetroot Almond Dip 110

Sour Cream...................................111

PASTA SAUCES

2 Ingredient Cooking Cream..........112

Creamy Capsicum Pasta 113

Mac 'n' Cheese 115

Creamy Mushroom Pasta 117

Basil Pesto 119

Alfredo Sauce 120

Walnut Pesto 122

SWEET TREATS

Cacao Bliss Balls............................123

Coconut Bliss Balls........................124

Mousse au Chocolate 125

Straw-Yo Pralines..........................126

Matcha Pralines.............................127

Choc-Yo Pralines...........................128

NICE CREAM & SMOOTHIES

Banana Nice Cream 129

Green Machine...............................130

Green Salted Caramel.....................131

Green Mango Lassi.........................132

Rich Chocolate Smoothie..............133

RECIPE LEGEND

🕐 Cook time

⧗ Wait time

🍴 Portions

MYLKS

How to Strain Mylk

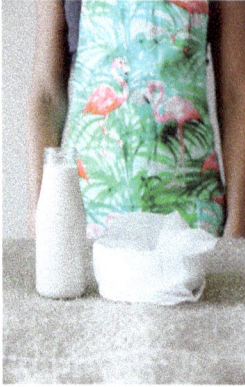

1. Put a nut mylk bag, fine sieve, thin tea towel or a cheese cloth into a bowl.

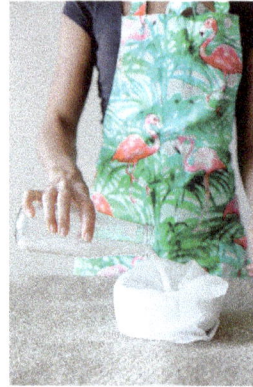

2. Pour the freshly blended mylk through the nut mylk bag into the bowl.

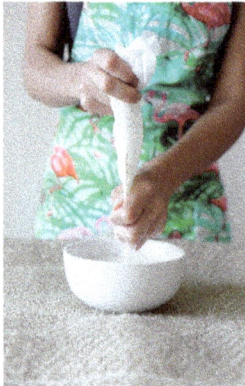

3. With your hands carefully squeeze out the remaining mylk.

Can you see the mylk splashing out? Mylk simply cannot be fresher!

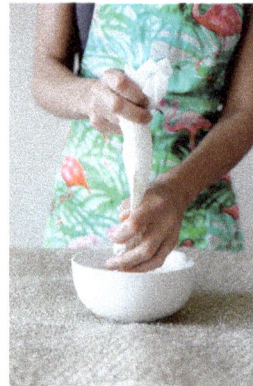

4. Once most of the liquid is squeezed out and the pulp is pretty dry, you can keep it, add it to smoothies, use it as almond flour for baking cookies etc.

BONUS: Check out *www.iquitdairy.com/bookbonus* and watch our short video on how to make your own mylk.

Kitchen hack

- You don't have to strain the mylk. In cereals and smoothies especially I leave it as is and enjoy the extra dose of fibre.

Cashew Mylk

🕐 5 mins   ⏳ 0 mins   🍴 2 cups

This mylk is ideal for coffee and tea as it doesn't split when you add it to hot beverages. Plus it is super smooth. Hands down this is my favourite mylk.

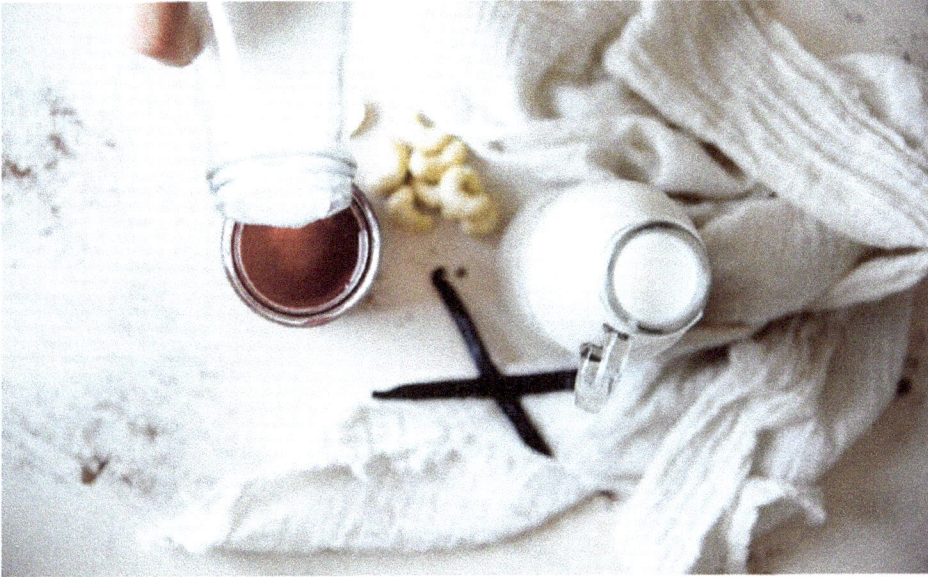

What's inside
- ⅓ cup raw cashews, soaked and drained
- 2 cups water
- 0.5 cm piece of vanilla bean / pinch of vanilla powder

How to
1. Add all the ingredients to a blender and blend until smooth (1-2 minutes).
2. Strain if you prefer.

Kitchen hack
- If you soak your cashews, you really don't have to strain this milk.

Almond Mylk

🕐 5 mins ⧗ 0 mins 🍴 2 cups

The mylk all-rounder. It has a nice taste and is so easy to make. This mylk just goes with pretty much any recipe and my go-to mylk for cereals.

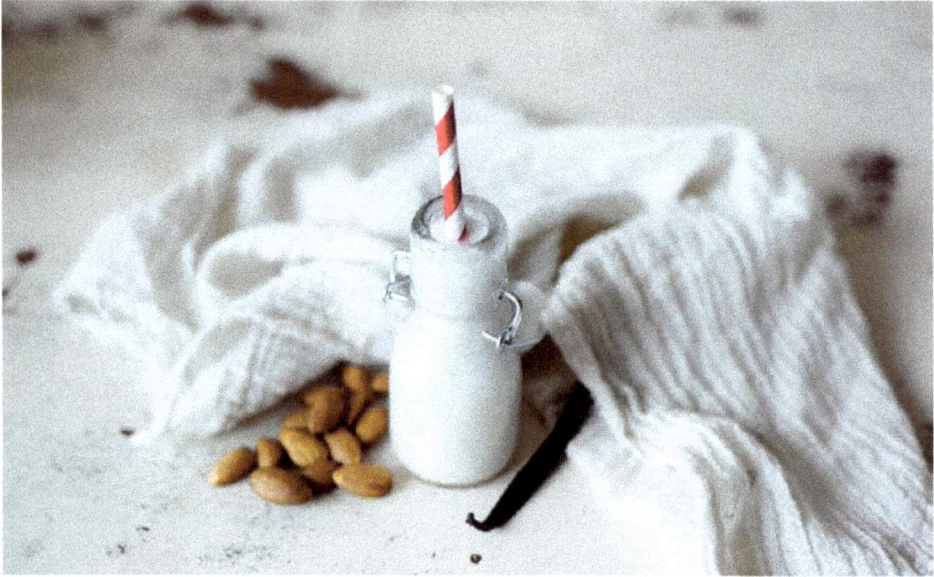

What's inside
- ⅓ cup almonds, soaked and drained
- 2 cups water
- 0.5 cm piece of vanilla bean / pinch of vanilla powder

How to
1. Add all the ingredients to a blender and blend until smooth (1-2 minutes).
2. Strain through a nut milk bag. I usually enjoy as is.

Kitchen hack
- In a rush? I occasionally skip the soaking and use activated almonds.
- Sweet-tooth? Simply add ½ a date. If it is too dry, soak it for 30 minutes.
- This milk is also great for smoothies. Instead of using store-bought milks, simply add water and nuts straight into the smoothie. This is better for both, your bank account and your body. Homemade mylks tend to be way cheaper than their convenient counterparts, plus they do not contain any nasties like sweeteners or thickeners.

Sunflower Seed Mylk

🕐 5 mins   ⧗ 0 mins   🍴 2 cups

A big surprise! I created this recipe for a course participant in our live events as her son is allergic to nuts. The taste really convinced me and the other participants alike. The date adds a yummy sweetness to the quite unique taste of this mylk. Worth trying.

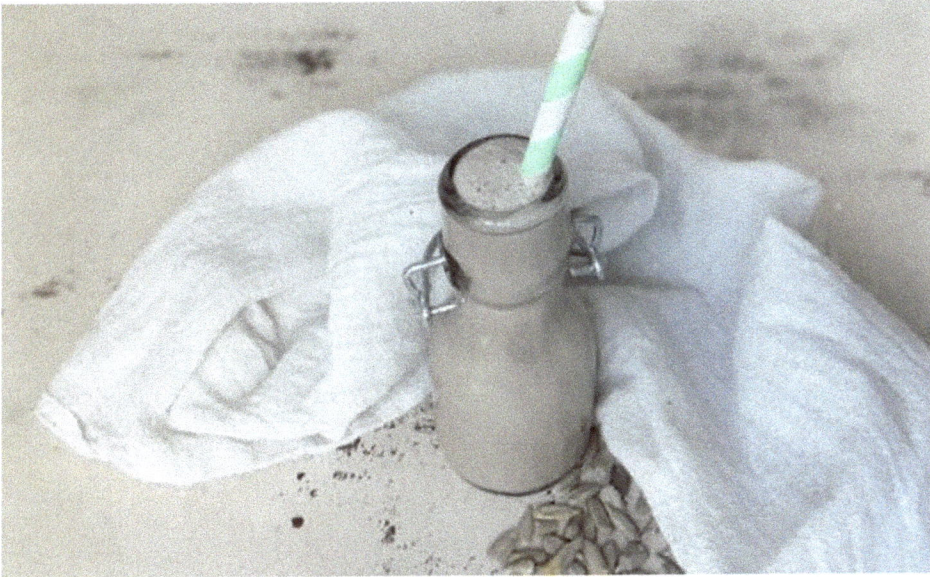

What's inside
- ⅓ cup sunflower seeds, soaked and drained
- 1 date, soaked
- 2 cups water

How to
1. Add all the ingredients to a blender and blend until smooth (1-2 minutes).
2. Strain through a nut milk bag.

Coconut Cream

🕐 5 mins   ⧗ 0 mins   🍴 2 cups

Goodbye canned coconut milk – hello REAL COCOMYLK. This cream is a true kitchen superstar. You can absolutely taste the difference and the best thing, you also get to drink the water while whipping it up. Who doesn't like to volunteer for this?

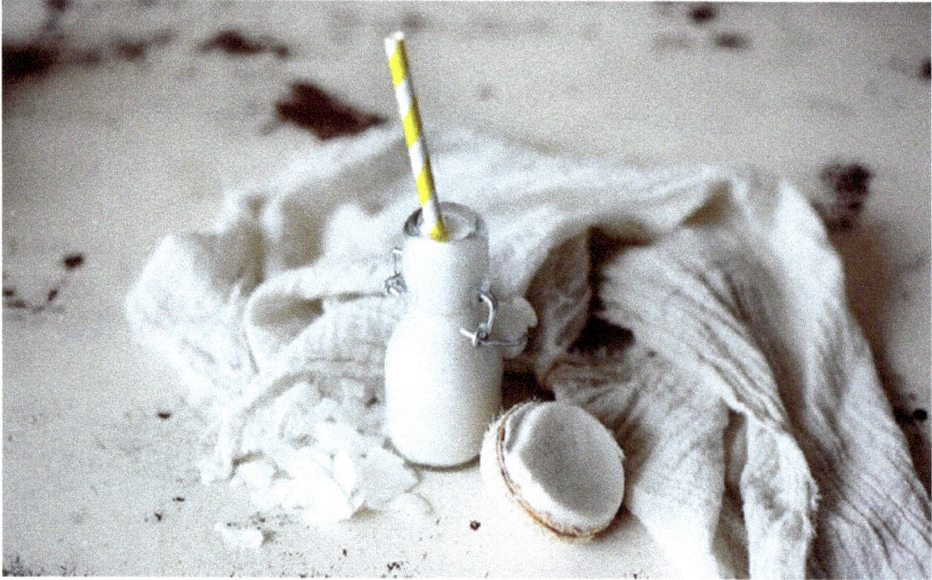

What's inside
- Meat of ½ a fresh coconut
- 2 cups water

How to
1. Add all the ingredients to a blender and blend until smooth (1-2 minutes).
2. Strain through a nut milk bag if you prefer.

Kitchen hack
- Taste the difference: Use this coconut cream in your next curry.
- To make coconut milk, simply dilute with 2 additional cups of water.
- The difference between coconut cream, milk and light is the water content. Often all three cost the same, so buy coconut cream. To turn a store-bought coconut cream into milk, simply mix it half and half with water. If you are after a light version, mix 3 parts water with 1 part coconut cream. Note every brand is a bit different.

Love Mylk

🕐 5 mins ⏳ 0 mins 🍴 2 cups

Thanks to the macadamias this mylk is rich and smooth in texture. The rose petals give it the extra hint of love and the lavender adds a beautiful sense of relaxation, all bound together with cardamom and cinnamon. A mylk you cannot get off the shelf.

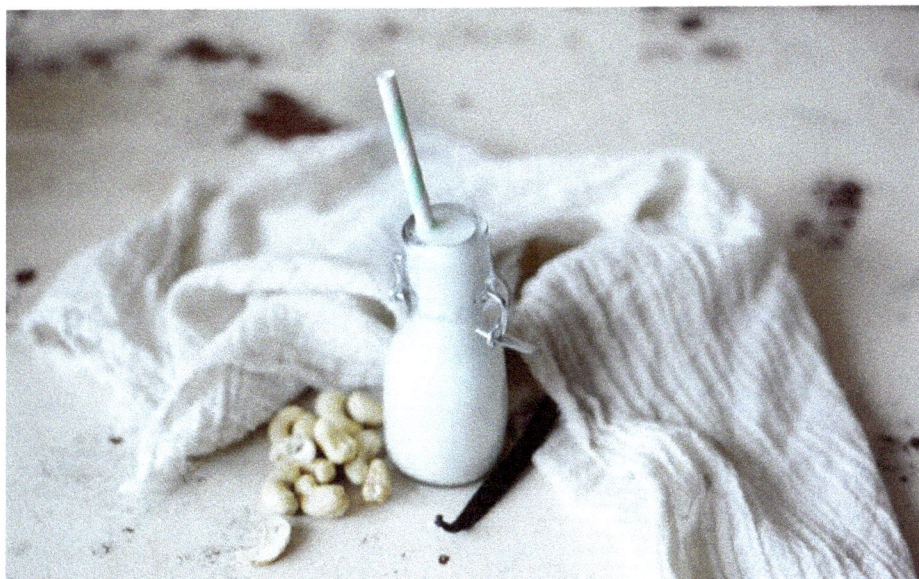

What's inside

- 2 cups water
- ¼ cup raw cashews, soaked and drained
- ¼ cup macadamia nuts, soaked
- 0.5 cm piece of vanilla bean
- ½ date
- some rose petals
- some dried lavender
- dash cardamom (optional)
- dash cinnamon (optional)

How to

1. First add water, nuts, vanilla bean and date to your blender and blend until you have a smooth, creamy milk. Depending on your blender it will take 20 seconds to 1 minute.
2. Strain if you prefer.
3. Return to your blender then add the remaining ingredients. Blend for another 20 seconds and enjoy.

Vanilla Brazil Mylk

🕐 5 mins ⏳ 0 mins 🍽 2 cups

On a nutrient side Brazil nuts are super high in selenium, which is good for our thyroid and therefore our hormones. Apart from that, this mylk is an absolute winner and it allows you to start experimenting with other nuts, than just the good-old Almond. Go kitchen angel, give it a go.

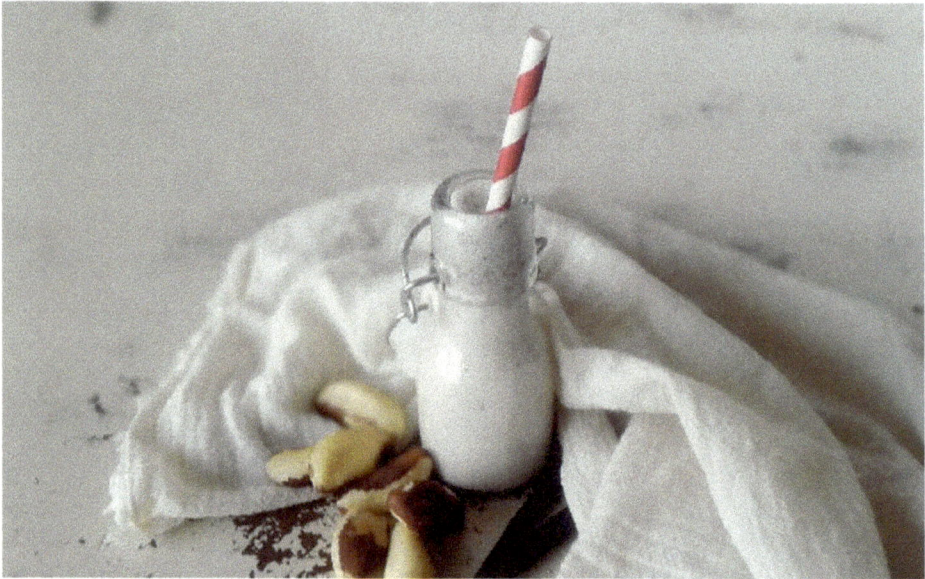

What's inside
- 2 cups water
- ⅓ cup Brazil nuts
- 2 cm vanilla pod

How to
1. Simply add everything to your blender and blend until you have a smooth, creamy milk. Depending on your blender it will take 20 seconds to 1 minute.
2. Strain if you prefer.

Deluxe Traveller's Mylk

🕐 5 mins   ⧗ 0 mins   🍴 1 cup

When I am travel, I always take some almond butter with me. It is the easiest mylk on earth, plus it adds a little morning work-out to your holidays. This mylk has already saved so many otherwise plain breakfasts for me.

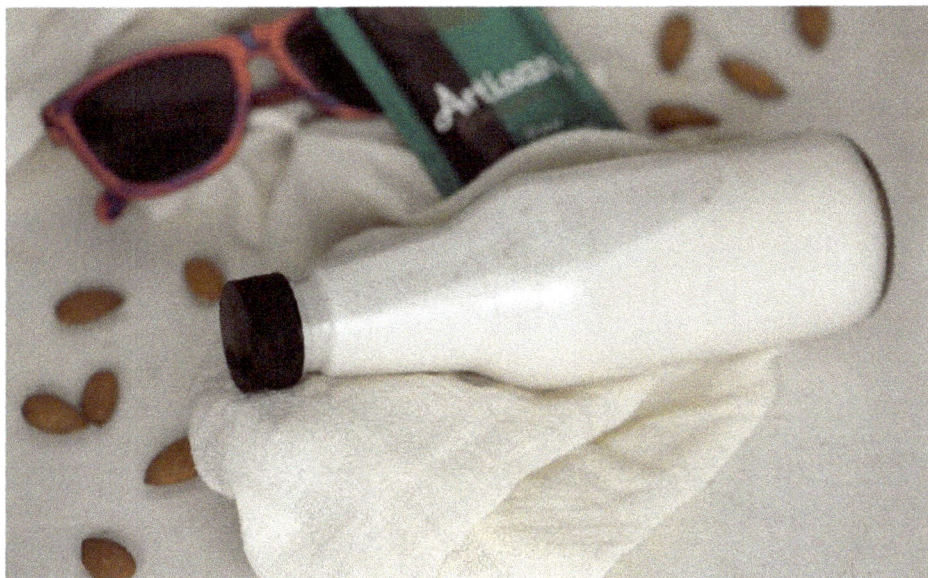

What's inside
- ½ a sachet almond butter (≈15g)
- 1 cup water

How to
1. Gently squeeze the closed sachet until the butter is nice and smooth.
2. Squeeze ½ of the nut butter into the bottle, filled with the water.
3. Shake the bottle until the butter is completely dissolved, et voilà the mylk is ready.

Variations
- You can use pretty much every nut butter and even coconut butter (not coconut oil).
- You can pimp the taste by adding spices like cinnamon or vanilla.
- If you have a sweet tooth you can of course also add a little bit of your preferred sweetener.

Buttermylk

🕐 10 mins   ⧗ 0 mins   🍴 1 cup

If you're a fan of buttermilk pancakes – this mylk is for you. I thought I had to give up on them but NO – this is the saviour. You can pretty much use any mylk. Bonsoy for example works really well, otherwise I usually use cashew mylk, just because of its creaminess.

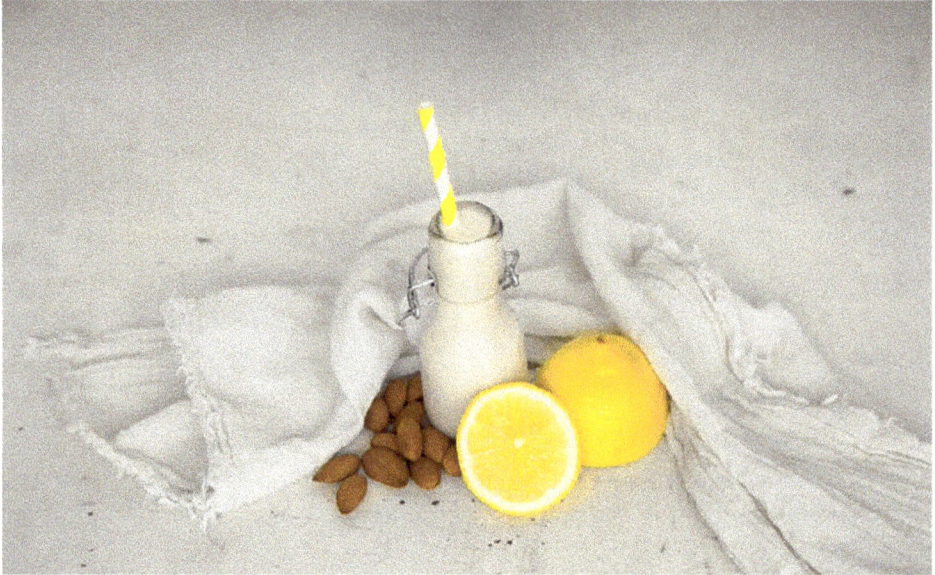

What's inside
- 1 cup mylk
- 1 Tbs lemon juice

How to
1. Combine the mylk with 1 tablespoon lemon juice.
2. Let stand for 5-10 minutes until the mylk has thickened.
3. Use as a replacement for buttermilk in your favourite recipes.

Pistachio Date Mylk

🕐 5 mins   ⧗ 0 mins   🍽 2 cups

I'm a creative! I love unleashing my creativity in the kitchen. I love colours, hence I had to come up with some colourful mylks, and this one is amazing. Yes, it involves a bit of work in case you first have to shell the pistachios by hand, but trust me it is absolutely worth it.

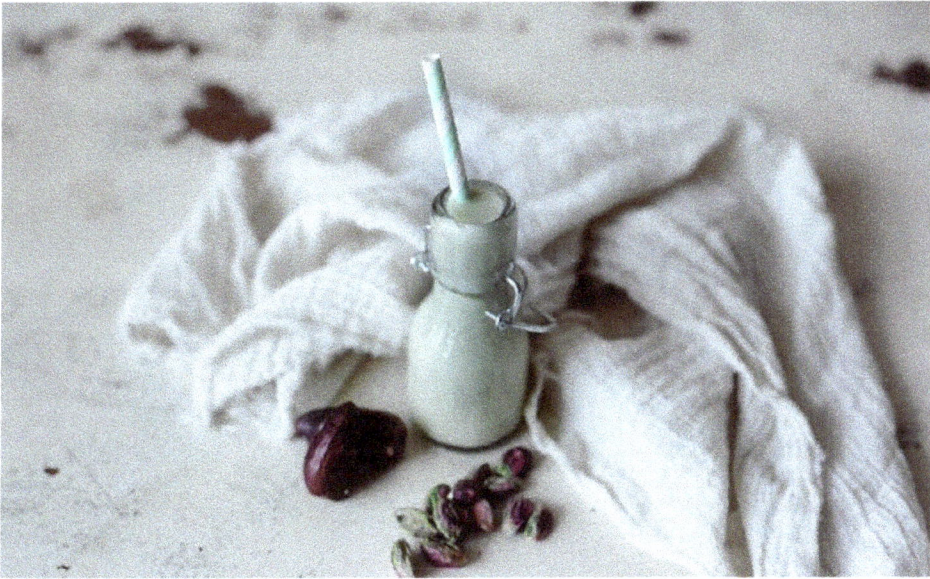

What's inside

- ⅓ cup raw shelled pistachios
- 1-2 cm vanilla bean or ½ tsp vanilla powder
- ½ a date, soaked
- 2 cups water

How to

1. Add all the ingredients to a blender and blend until smooth (1-2 minutes).
2. Strain through a nut milk bag.

Kitchen hack

- To get a really green milk you need to shell the pistachios. The easiest way to do this is to soak the pistachios for 2-3 hours. As the nut skin gets softer you can easily peel it off with your hands.

Macadamia Orange Mylk

🕐 5 mins   ⌛ 0 mins   🍽 2 cups

Where there is green pistachio mylk – orange has to follow. Check out this macadamia orange mylk – all I want to say is #nom! The creaminess of the macadamia goes so well with the soft flavour of the orange zest.

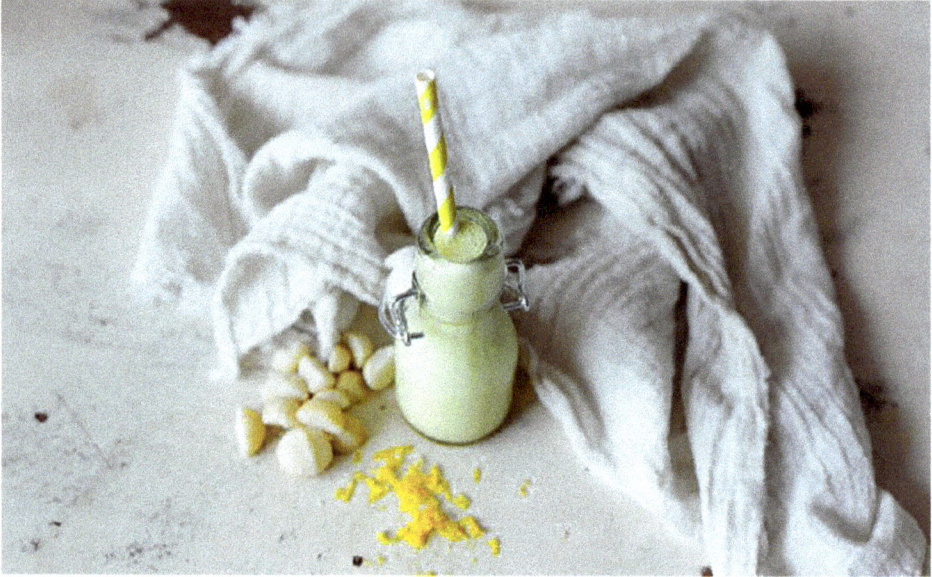

What's inside
- ⅓ cup macadamias, soaked and drained
- Zest of ½ an organic orange
- 2 cups water

How to
1. Blend until smooth (1-2 minutes).
2. Strain through a nut milk bag.

Kitchen hack
- Macadamia milk is maybe the smoothest self-made mylk you can make. It's ideal for puddings or vanilla sauce, so creamy.

Chocolate Hazelmylk

🕐 5 mins   ⏳ 0 mins   🍴 2 cups

Where there is mylk – there has to be chocolate. This recipe is the adult version of a rich chocolate drink. The combination of cloves, vanilla and cinnamon are a match made in heaven – pure indulgence, just healthy.

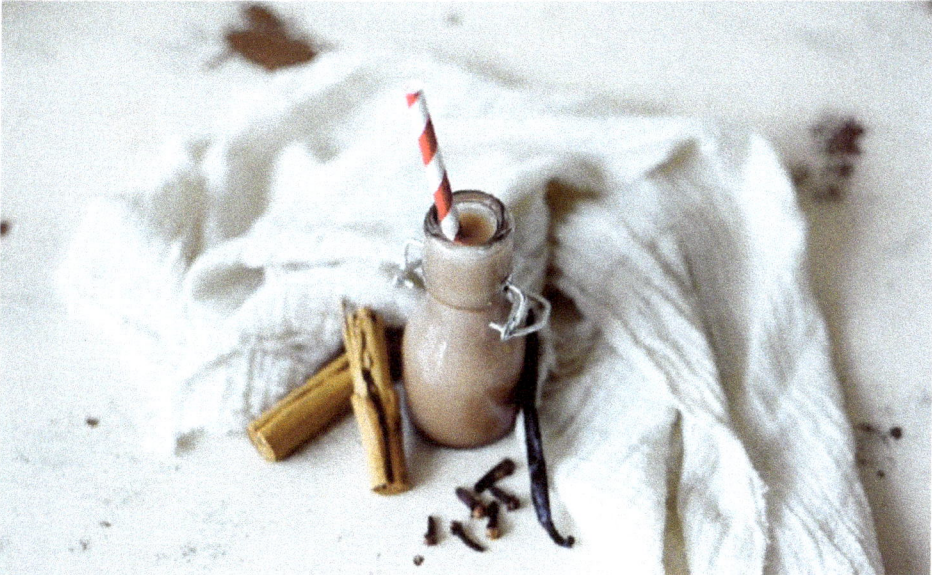

What's inside

- ⅓ cup (1 handful) hazelnuts, soaked and drained
- 2 cups water
- 1 tsp cacao
- 1 tsp maple syrup
- Pinch of vanilla
- Pinch of cloves
- Pinch of cinnamon

How to

1. Add all the ingredients to a blender and blend until smooth (1-2 minutes).
2. Strain if you prefer. I love it rich with everything still in it.

BREAKFAST

Everyday Cereals

🕐 10 mins   ⧗ 0 mins   🍽 6

I always have a jar of this cereal in the pantry. Add your favourite fruit and move with the season to make this a quick year-round yummy breakfast.

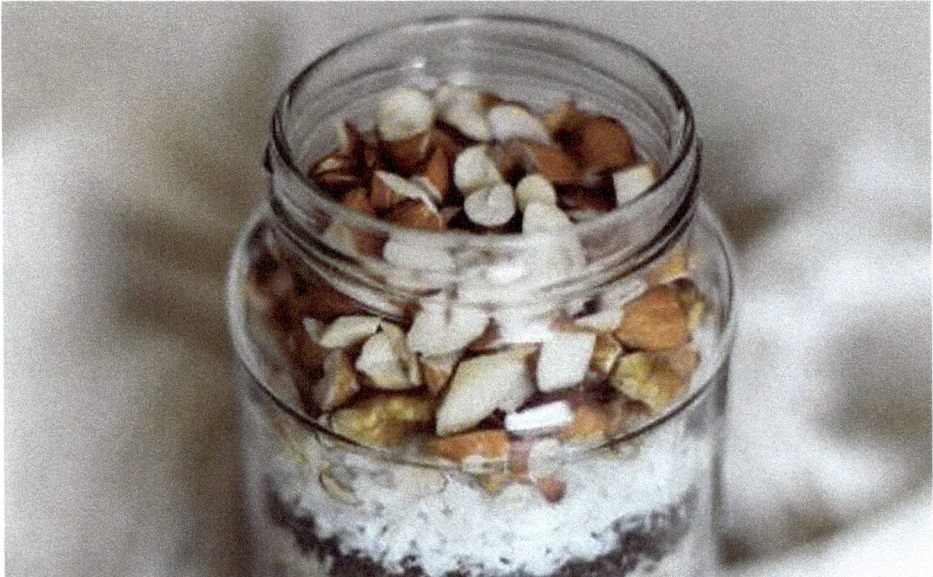

What's inside
- ½ cup popped quinoa
- ½ cup popped amaranth
- ¼ cup sunflower seeds
- ¼ cup sunflower pepitas
- ¼ cup sesame seeds
- ¼ cup chia seeds
- ⅓ cup walnuts, chopped
- ⅓ cup almonds, chopped
- ⅓ cup unsweetened shredded coconut flakes
- ¼ tsp vanilla powder

How to
1. Add all the ingredients to a jar and shake until everything is well combined.

2. For breakfast, simply combine ½ a cup of cereal with ½ a cup of fresh seasonal fruits (like blueberries, apples, strawberries, bananas, watermelon or passionfruit) and your favourite nut milk.

Swaps

- You can also add oats, raw buckwheat or sugar-free cornflakes.

Power Porridge

🕐 15 mins　　⧗ 0 mins　　🍴 2

The winter warmer. In the colder months I often feel like a nice warm breakfast. The beauty of this one is that it is super quick and filled with heaps of energy to kick-start you into the day.

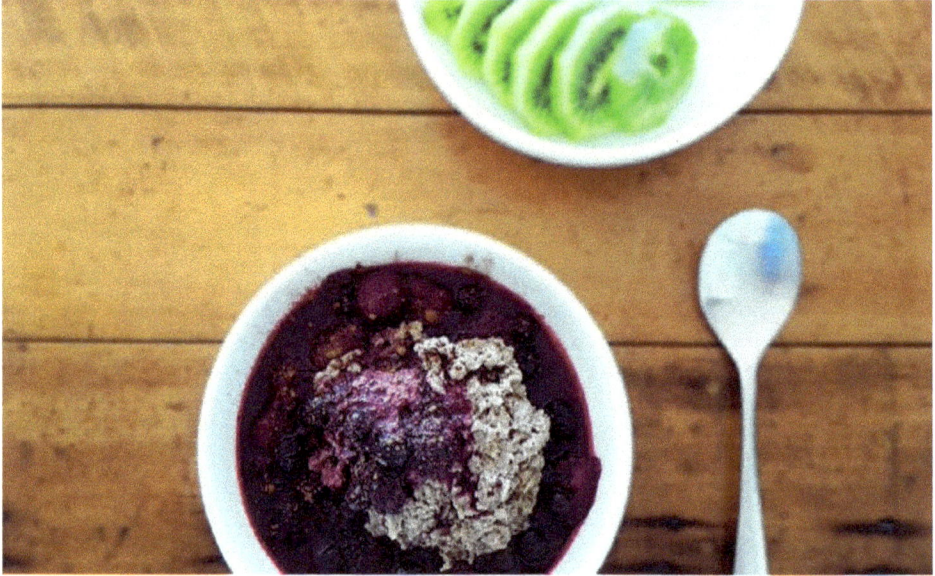

What's inside

- ½ cup gluten-free oats
- 1 ½ cups water
- ¼ cup walnuts, roughly cut
- 1 Tbs chia seeds
- 1 Tbs shredded coconut
- 1 Tbs buckwheat
- 1 Tbs sunflower seeds
- 1 Tbs pepitas
- 1 Tbs hemp seeds (optional)
- 1 cup frozen mixed berries
- ¼ cup water

How to

1. Cook oats with water on medium heat in a pot with the lid closed for about 10 minutes until soft. Stir occasionally so the mixture doesn't stick or burn.
2. Meanwhile in a separate pot warm the frozen berries with water. If you like, add some cinnamon and vanilla.

3. Mix the walnuts, chia seeds, coconut, raw buckwheat, sunflower seeds and pepitas, and stir half of the mix through the porridge once ready.
4. Divide the berries and power porridge between 2 breakfast bowls.

Swaps
- Rolled Oats from the brands Bob's Red Mill and Glorious Foods are considered gluten-free in Europe and the US.
- If you cannot tolerate oats simply replace with quinoa flakes or use a mix of ¼ cup buckwheat kernels and ¼ cup sunflower seeds.

Chia Pudding with Apple Sauce

🕐 5 mins ⧗ 2 hrs 🍴 1

When I first went dairy-free I hadn't heard of chia seeds, now I cannot live without them. You can have this for breakfast or dessert. It is super easy and really versatile. Sss You can play around with different flavours, like add some acai powder or different spices. Experiment and see what your favourite is.

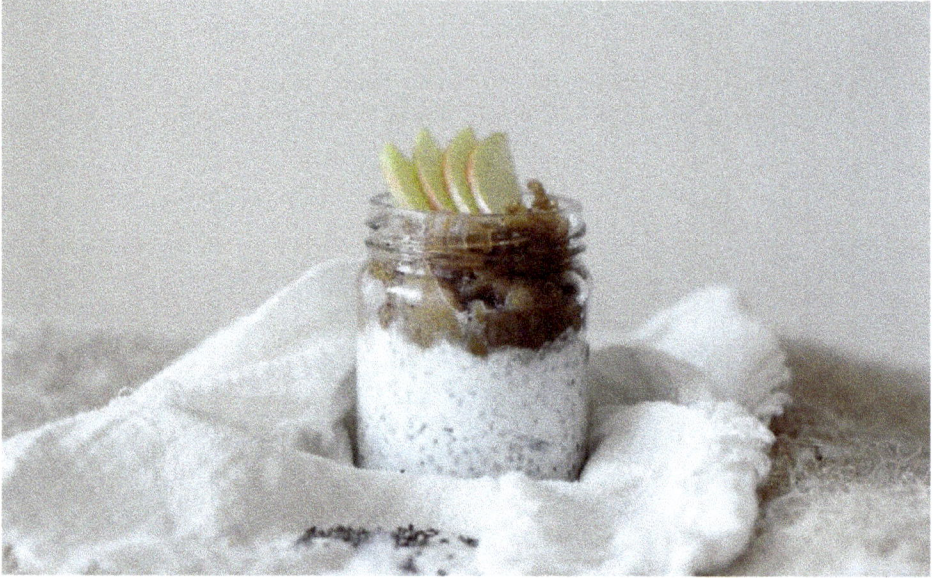

What's inside

- 1 Tbs chia seeds
- ⅓ cup of your favourite mylk
- 1 pinch of vanilla powder
- Fresh fruit or apple sauce

How to

1. Combine the chia seeds, coconut milk and vanilla powder in a jar. Close, mix well and refrigerate overnight.
2. In the morning, top it up with some fresh fruits or homemade apple sauce.

Kitchen hack

- If you use frozen fruit, add the fruit directly to the coconut-chia mix, so it can defrost as well.

Chocolate Overnight Oats

🕐 5 mins   ⧖ 4 hrs   🍴 2

The perfect on-the-go brekkie and recipe favourite in our I Quit Dairy live events. We usually get photos in the following days with beautiful re-creations.

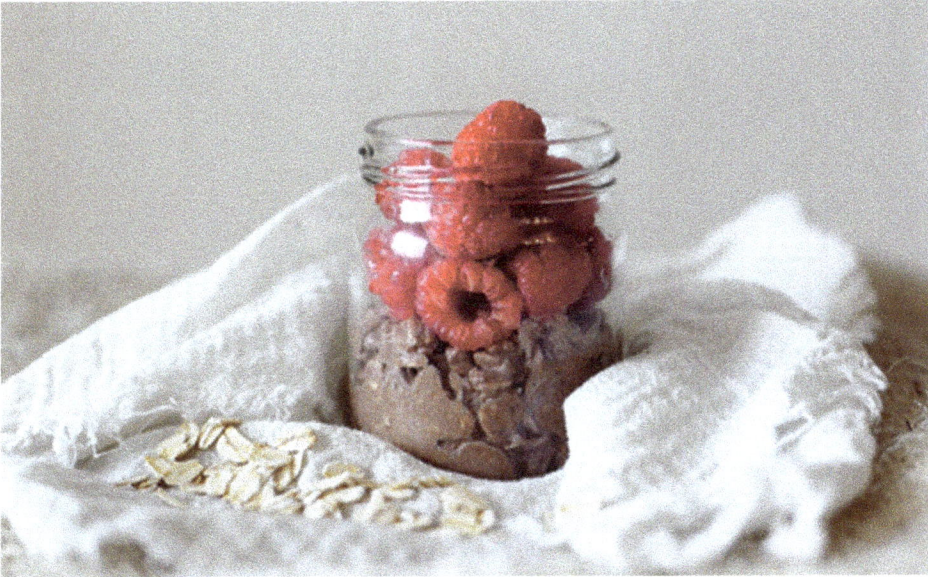

What's inside
- ½ a large banana
- ¼ cup mylk or water
- ½ cup gluten-free oats
- 4 tsp cacao
- Fresh fruit (like blueberries)

How to
1. Mash the banana with a fork.
2. Place the banana, mylk, oats and cacao into a bowl and mix until everything is well combined. Fill a jar with the mixture and refrigerate overnight.
3. In the morning add fruits on top and enjoy!

Kitchen hack
- If you use frozen fruit, add the fruit in the evening to defrost.

Swaps
- Rolled oats from the brands Bob's Red Mill and Glorious Foods are considered gluten-free in Europe and the US.
- If you cannot tolerate oats simply replace with quinoa flakes or use a mix of ¼ cup buckwheat kernels and ¼ cup sunflower seeds.
- For a richer version you can replace the mylk with dairy-free yogurt.

Peach Melba Overnight Oats

🕐 5 mins   ⏳ 4 hrs   🍴 2

Being a busy business woman, I know how precious time is, especially in the morning. I set time aside to meditate and exercise and then I love to simply open the fridge and have yummy and nourishing food waiting for me. If you're like me—give it a try.

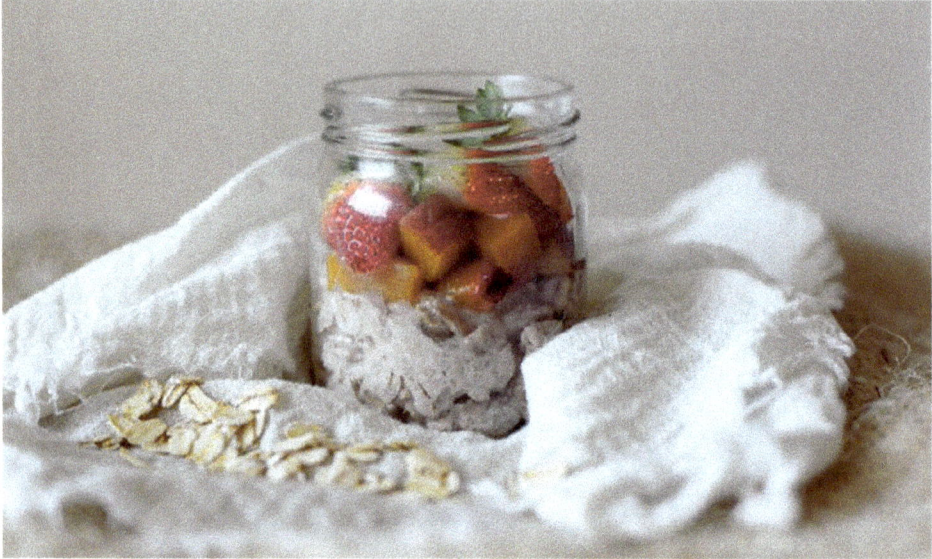

What's inside

- ½ large banana
- ¼ cup of your favourite mylk or water
- ½ cup gluten-free oats
- 1 tsp vanilla
- ½ tsp cinnamon
- Fresh fruit (like peaches or raspberries)

How to

1. Mash the banana with a fork.
2. Place the banana, mylk, oats, vanilla and cinnamon into a bowl and mix until everything is well combined. Fill a jar with the mix and refrigerate overnight.
3. In the morning add fruits on top and enjoy!

Kitchen hack

- If you use frozen fruit, add the fruit directly to the oat mix to defrost.

Swaps

- Rolled Oats from the brands Bob's Red Mill and Glorious Foods are considered gluten-free in Europe and the US.
- If you cannot tolerate oats simply replace with quinoa flakes or use a mix of ¼ cup buckwheat kernels and ¼ cup sunflower seeds.
- For a richer version you can replace the mylk with dairy-free yogurt.

Superpower Breakfast Smoothie

🕐 5 mins ⏳ 0 mins 🍴 2

Sometimes I don't feel like chewing and I want something on the go. Smoothies are just perfect for this. Plus chocolate for breakfast is just such a sweet start to the day :)

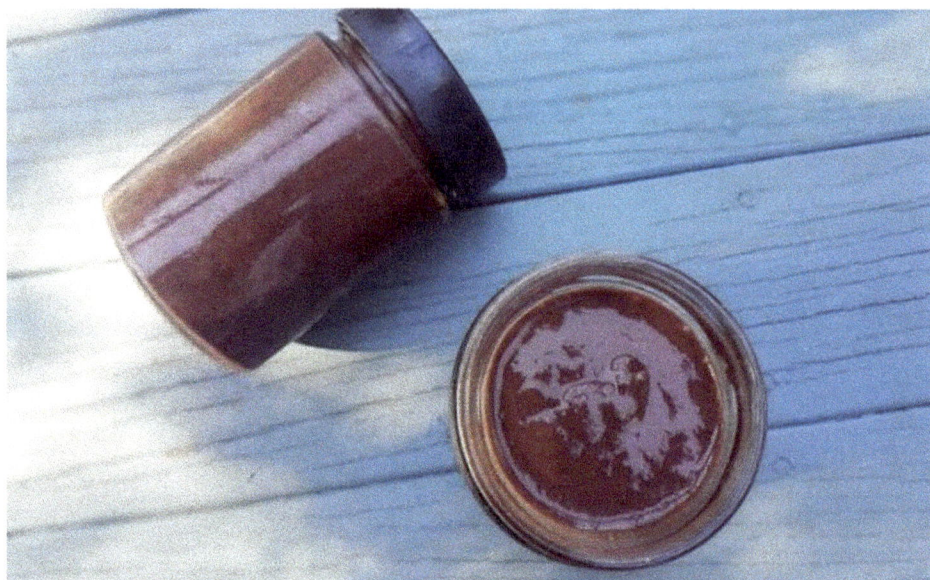

What's inside

- ½ cup coconut water
- ¼ cup water
- 1 cup spinach
- 1 frozen banana
- ¼ cup frozen blue berries

- 2 Tbs cacao powder
- 2 Tbs flaxseeds
- ¼ cup gluten-free oats
- 1 tsp slippery elm
- ¼ cup almonds

How to

1. Add everything to your blender, liquids first.
2. Blend until smooth.

Swaps

- Rolled Oats from the brands Bob's Red Mill and Glorious Foods are considered gluten-free in Europe and the US.
- If you cannot tolerate oats simply replace with quinoa flakes or use a mix of ¼ cup buckwheat kernels and ¼ cup sunflower seeds.

Açai Bowl

🕐 5 mins   ⧗ 0 mins   🍽 2

WOW! Who doesn't love açai bowls – they are the most perfect and prettiest way to start your day. When I was in Brazil—the home of açai—I was amazed at how prominent they were, and eating a bowl on top of the Sugarloaf was maybe the most exotic place I've ever had one. Just imagine travelling and everywhere you can buy one of these beautiful and nourishing bowls = dairy-free paradise!

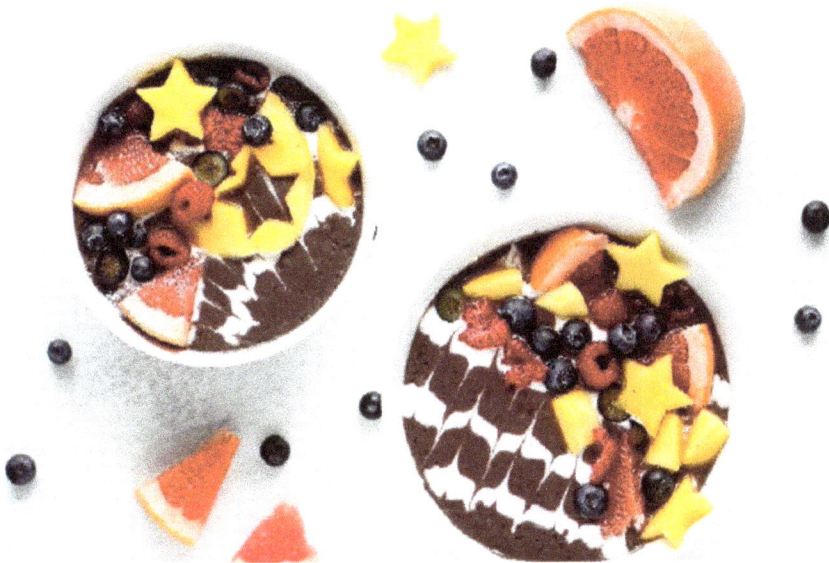

What's inside

- 1/3 cup coconut water or water
- 1 frozen banana, peeled and cut into pieces
- ½ cup spinach
- 1 pack frozen açai puree
- Fresh fruits or granola for decoration

How to

1. Add all the ingredients to your blender and blend.
2. Occasionally turn the blender off and scrape down the fruit until you get a smooth texture. This might take about 2 minutes (depending on your blender).
3. Decorate with fresh fruit or granola and enjoy!

Ultimate Banana Yogurt

🕐 5 mins ⏳ 0 mins 🍴 2

This breakfast brings back so many wonderful childhood memories. Back then one of my favourite snacks was bananas with yogurt. I would always mash the bananas with a fork in the yogurt and this recipe tastes exactly like my self-made creation. Yum!

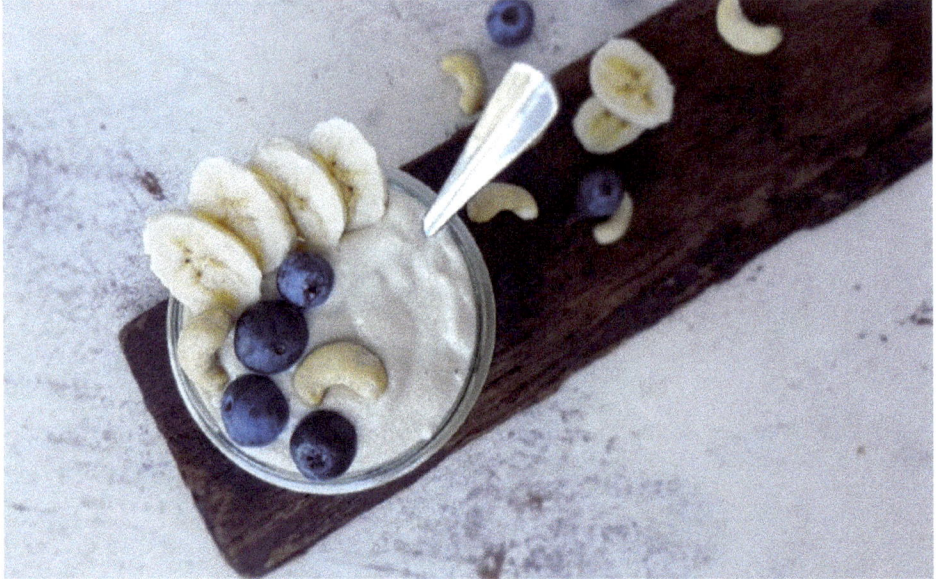

What's inside
- 2 bananas
- 2/3 cup cashews, soaked and drained
- ¼ cup coconut water
- 2 Tbs lemon juice (½ lemon)
- 1 pinch salt
- 1 punnet blueberries

How to
1. Add 1 banana with the other ingredients to a blender and blend until smooth (1-2 mins).
2. Occasionally turn the blender off and scrape down the sauce until you get a smooth texture. This will take about 1-2 minutes.
3. While the blender is running, slice the banana and wash the blueberries.
4. Divide the yogurt into two bowls and decorate with the fruit.

Power Granola

🕐 10 mins 　⧖ 10 mins 　🍴 1.5 cups

A little treat and the hubby loves it. The granola works perfectly with açai bowls and cereals. It is also a great companion with desserts. Try it.

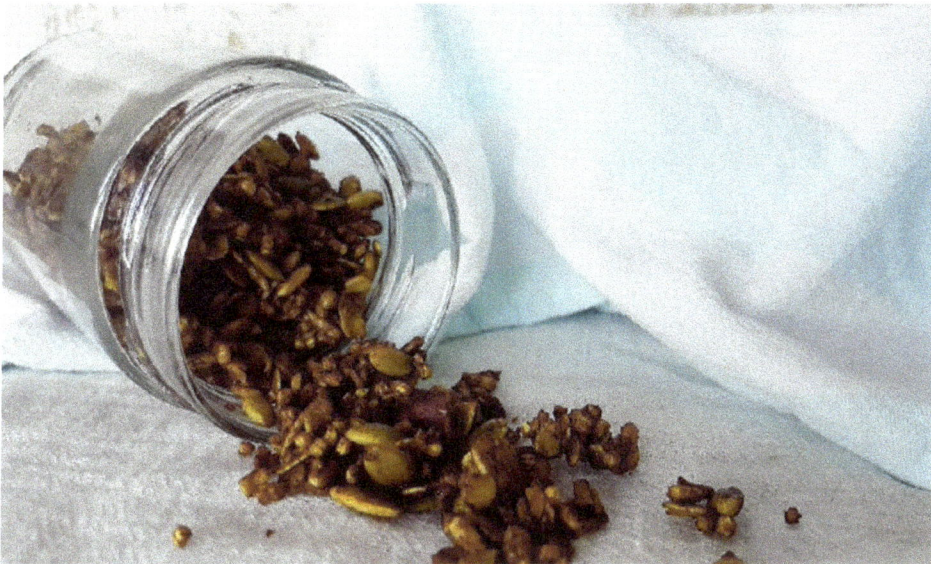

What's inside

- ½ cup gluten-free oats
- ¼ cup sunflower seeds
- ¼ cup pepitas
- ¼ cup puffed quinoa
- ¼ cup puffed amaranth
- 2 Tbs coconut sugar
- 2 Tbs coconut oil
- ½ tsp cinnamon powder
- ½ tsp pumpkin pie spice

How to

1. Preheat the oven to 180C.
2. In a medium bowl combine all ingredients until everything is well coated.
3. Spread evenly on a lined baking tray.
4. Bake for 10 minutes or until crisp and golden. Check every now and then to make sure the granola bakes evenly. Gently mix if required.
5. Once the granola is done, take it out of the oven and let cool. Store in an airtight container or immediately add to your breakfast or dessert.

Swaps

- Swap the oats for quinoa flakes or coconut shreds if you prefer.
- Be creative with the spices and try different flavours. cinnamon, nutmeg, vanilla, ginger, cardamom, cloves and turmeric are beautiful flavours.
- For an oil-free version: You can swap the oil for 2 Tbs of apple sauce (ideally self-made, without added sugars).

Pumpkin Pancake

🕐 10 mins   ⏳ 0 mins   🍴 2

No more pancakes? Ha, not in my world. I do love pancakes and these ones are delicious plus you can whip up the batter in your blender. They're even gluten-free and work for both sweet and savoury creations.

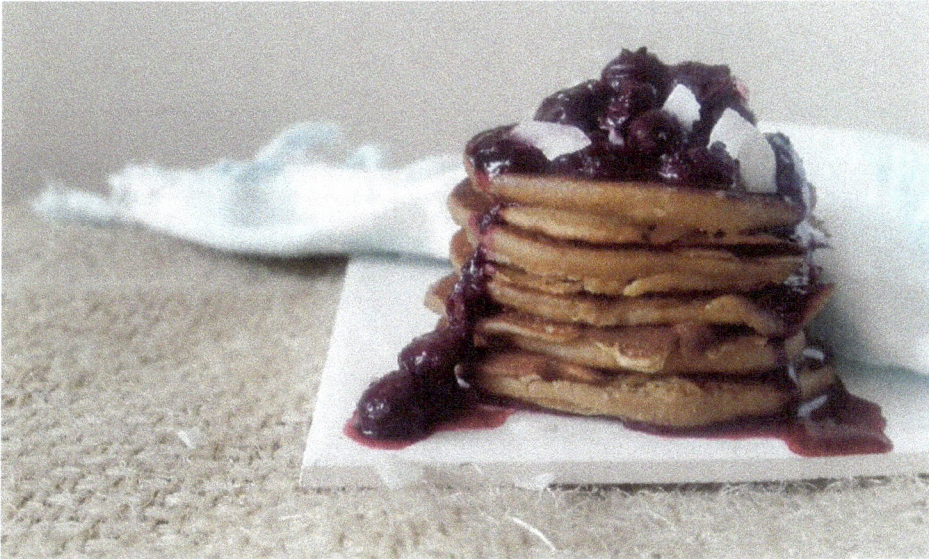

What's inside

- 1 cup rice mylk
- 2 Tbs pumpkin purée (leftover roasted pumpkin)
- ½ cup quinoa or millet flour
- ¼ cup macadamia nuts (or cashews/almonds)
- 1 cm vanilla bean (or ½ tsp vanilla powder)
- 2 tsp pumpkin pie spice
- 1 banana, sliced
- 1 punnet fresh organic blueberries

How to

1. Add all the ingredients except the banana and blueberries to your food processor.
2. Preheat a non-stick pan to medium/hot.
3. Blend the batter in your food processor and check the consistency. It should be a like a traditional pancake batter – not too runny and not to firm – adjust with water as needed.

4. Carefully pour the batter into the pan, forming little pancakes.
5. As soon as little air bubbles appear on the top side of your pancakes, they are asking to be turned. Be soft and gentle. Turn them with love.
6. Keep the pancakes warm in the oven at 50°C until all pancakes are done.
7. Stack the pancakes and decorate with fresh banana slices and blueberries.
8. To finish sprinkle some cinnamon on top of the pancakes and enjoy.

Variations

The job of the rice milk is to add a little natural sweetness. If you don't have any handy, simply replace with 1 cup of water.

- These pancakes are the perfect match for my dairy-free Acai Ice Dream. Who doesn't love pancakes and ice cream for breakfast?
- If you don't have any fresh fruit, simply make this

Quick and Easy sugar-free Blueberry Sauce:

1. Add 1 cup frozen blueberries and ¼ cup water to a pot and heat on a low heat.
2. Stir occasionally until the fruit gets soft and the sauce thickens up a bit. It should be a rich and naturally sweet sauce, which will perfectly soak into the pancakes and make them look even better.

Smooth Coco Chai Quinoa

🕐 20 mins ⏳ 0 mins 🍴 4

I love preparing this for our camping trips. I cook up a big batch and put it in our camping fridge. That way we have a yummy and filling breakfast for the first few days without any cooking.

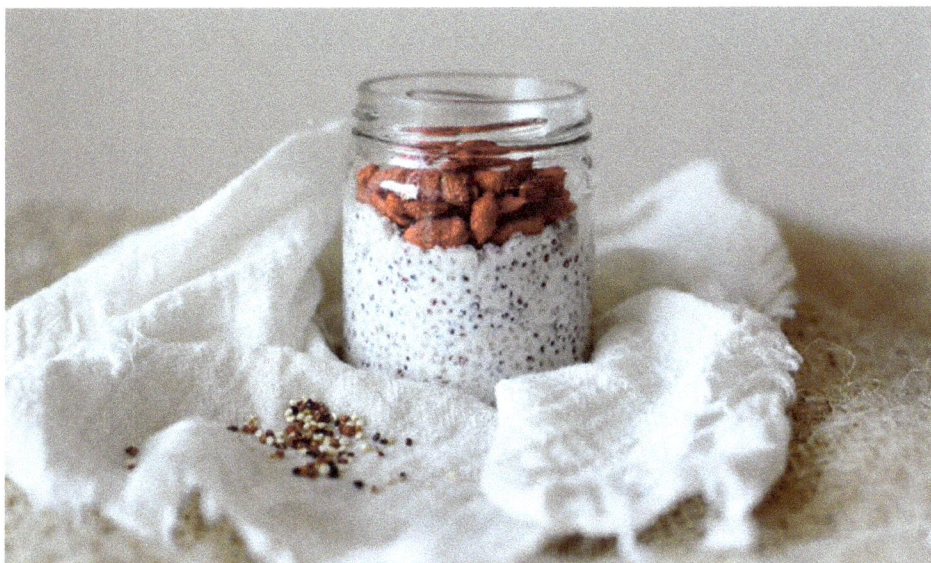

What's inside

- ½ cup quinoa
- 1 cup of your favourite mylk
- ½ cup water
- ½ tsp cinnamon
- ¼ tsp cardamom
- ¼ tsp vanilla powder
- A dash of nutmeg
- ½ cup coconut yogurt
- Some fresh fruit

How to

1. Place the quinoa in a fine-mesh strainer and rinse well with cold water.
2. Add all the ingredients into a pot. Heat up and bring to the boil. Reduce to low-medium heat and cover with a lid. Leave to simmer for roughly 15 minutes until all the liquid has been absorbed.
3. Discard the spices and either put the mix straight into a bowl with some fruits or use it to fill a container and store in the fridge until breakfast time.
4. Mix the quinoa with the yogurt, add your favourite fruits and enjoy your breakfast.

Kitchen hack

- If you just have coconut cream use ½ cup coconut cream and ½ cup water.
- Eat it straight away for breakfast or store it in an airtight container in the fridge for a couple of days.

Swaps

- For an oil-free version: Swap the coconut yogurt for soy or nut-based yogurt or some mashed banana or pumpkin puree.

Filling Real Fruit Yogurt

🕐 5 mins ⏳ 0 mins 🍴 2 cups

I have done my own fruit yogurts for ages. Years back food investigators found actual pieces of wood in strawberry yogurts which were meant to make the consumer believe they were strawberry bits. I couldn't ignore that. I started checking the amount of fruit in yogurts and realised that it was close to nothing, so this is a delicious and quick alternative.

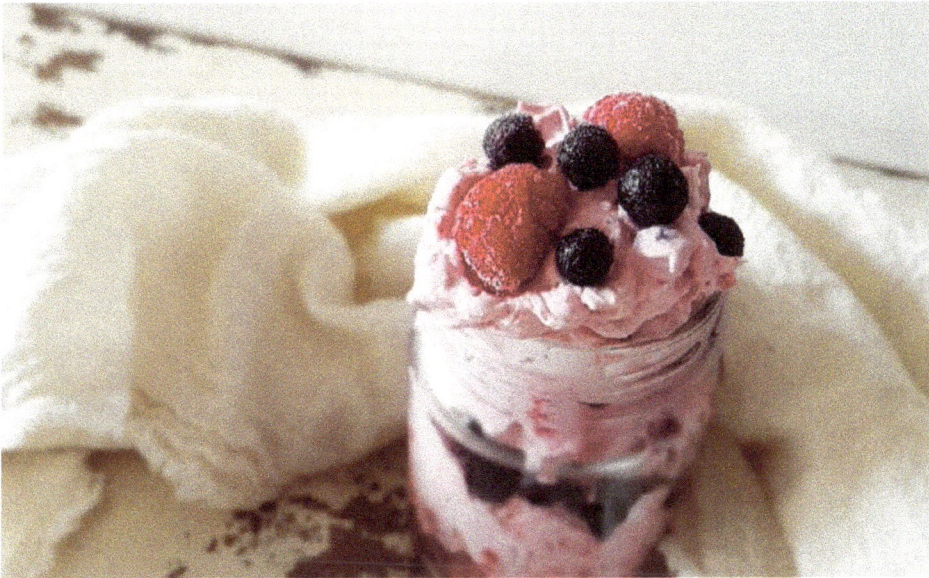

What's inside
- ¼ cup dairy-free yogurt (like coconut or soy yogurt)
- 1 Tbs gluten-free oats
- 2 Tbs frozen fruit

How to
1. Simply mix the yogurt and oats with a spoon.
2. Fold in the fruits and leave in the fridge for 1-2 hours, or overnight to allow the fruit to defrost.

Swap
- Rolled Oats from the brands Bob's Red Mill and Glorious Foods are considered gluten-free in Europe and the US.
- If you cannot tolerate oats simply replace with quinoa flakes, buckwheat kernels or sunflower seeds.

CHEESES

Parmesan

🕐 5 mins   ⏳ 0 mins   🍴 1/2 cup

For all the Bolognese lovers out there this 5 ingredients parmesan is an absolute life saver. Thanks to the nutritional yeast the flavour gets really cheesy! I blend up a batch and store it in a jar in the fridge and it lasts forever.

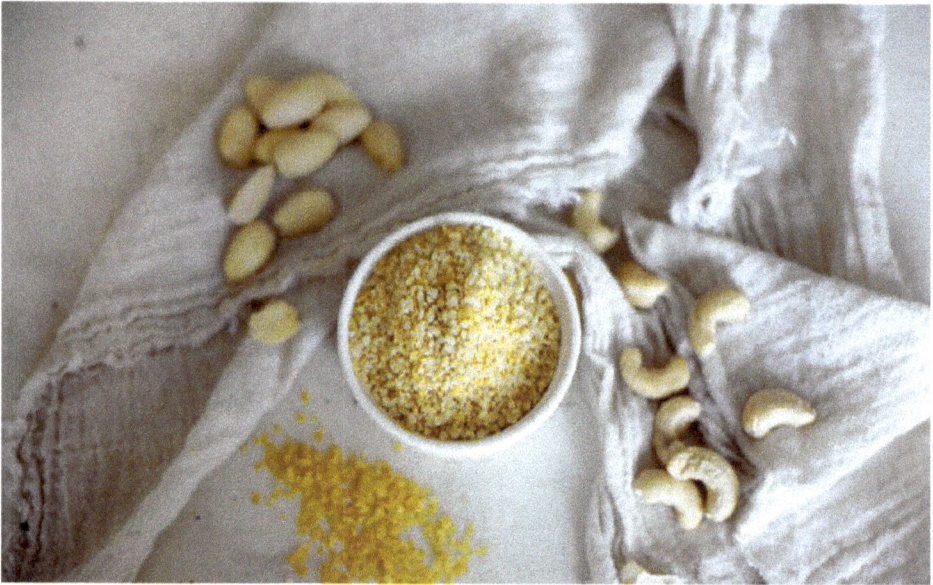

What's inside
- ¼ cup blanched almonds
- ¼ cup raw cashews
- 1 Tbs + 2 tsp nutritional yeast
- ½ tsp sea salt
- ¼ tsp garlic powder

How to
1. Add all the ingredients to your food processor and pulse for a few seconds until everything is well combined and still crumbly.
2. Don't blend for too long, or the parmesan will turn into a nut butter.

Crumbly Macadamia Cheeze

🕐 10 mins   ⏳ 0 mins   🍴 1/2 cup

This cheeze is the perfect match for a traditional rocket, pear and walnut salad. Whipped up in less than a few minutes. The combination of salt and lemon gives it a distinct tangy taste.

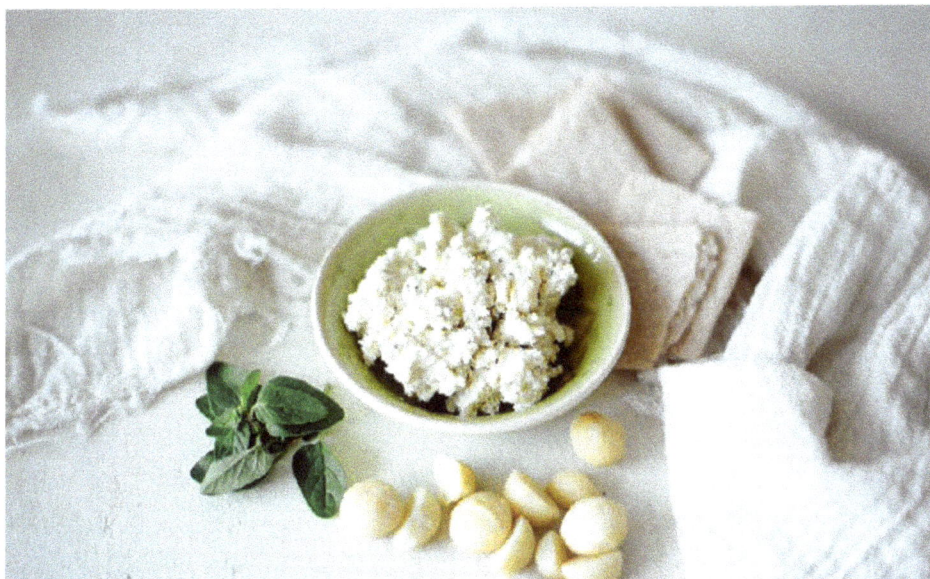

What's inside

- 1 Tbs water (add more if desired)
- ½ cup macadamias, soaked and drained
- 1 Tbs nutritional yeast
- Pinch of sea salt
- 1 Tbs lemon juice (¼ a lemon)

How to

1. Add all the ingredients to your food processor and pulse a couple of times for a few seconds until nice and crumbly.
2. Check the taste and add more lemon if you prefer a tangier taste, or water for a runnier consistency. Once it's perfect, simply scrape it out and crumble on top of your favourite salad.

Herbed Cheeze Wheel

🕐 20 mins ⏳ 12-48 hrs 🍴 1

This recipe is for the slightly advanced dairy-free heroes. It's my absolute favourite cashew cheeze and all my friends, even the cheese addicts, love it. So be gutsy and give it a go.

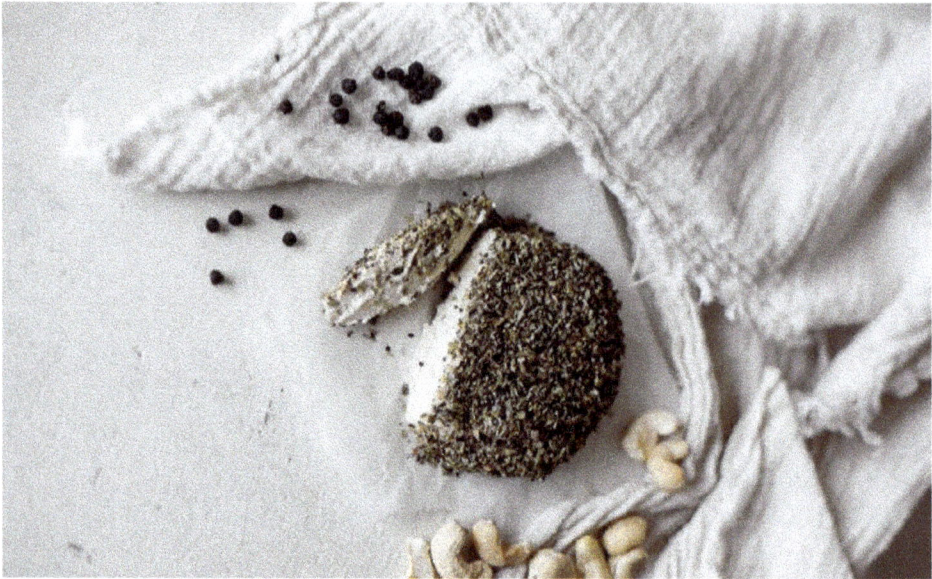

What's inside

- ⅓ cup water
- 1 cup cashews, soaked and drained
- ½ garlic clove
- ½ lemon, zested and juiced (4 Tbs)
- 1 Tbs nutritional yeast
- ¼ tsp sea salt

Decoration

- 1 Tbs cracked pepper
- 2 tsp dried oregano
- 2 tsp dried basil
- 2 tsp dried thyme

How to

1. Add all the ingredients to your blender and blend.
2. Occasionally turn the blender off and scrape down the cheese until you get a smooth texture. This will take about 2-3 minutes.
3. Lay a cheesecloth (or other muslin cloth, like a thin tea towel) in a bowl.

4. Pour the mixture into the centre of the cheesecloth. Close the cheesecloth with a rubber band and hang the cheese above a bowl so that excess water can drain out.

5. Leave the cheese in the cloth for at least 12 hours (ideally 24-48 hours) – the longer the rest time, the firmer the cheese.

6. Check if the cheese is ready by opening the cheesecloth. If it stays the same shape and you can see the structure of the cheesecloth then it is dry enough; if the cheese 'melts' or is still runny, it needs some more time.

7. In a small bowl mix the pepper and herbs.

8. To wrap the cheese in its herbed crust, put the cheese in the cheesecloth on a board. Open the cheesecloth on all sides, leaving the cheese ball in the middle. Carefully form the desired shape by pressing it a down little bit until you get the typical flat, round cheese shape. Evenly spread out 1 tablespoon of the pepper-herbs mix on the cheesecloth next to one side of the cheese. With great care using the cheesecloth, turn the cheese onto the herbed side. Continue this strategy until the whole cheese is covered and finish by decorating on a nice board.

Kitchen hack

-   Instead of hanging the cheese you can also put the cheese mixture in the cheesecloth in a sieve on top of a bowl and add some weights (like one or two cans) on top to squeeze out the excess liquid.

-   If your cheese doesn't get firm enough you have a couple of options:
    1. Leave it in the fridge for a bit longer.
    2. Transfer it to a thinner muslin.
    3. Squeeze out some of the water by hand.

Melting Pizza Cheeze

🕐 20 mins ⏳ 0 mins 🍴 1 cup

Thought you would never have any nice gooey cheese again? Try this one. I really love this melting cheese on pizza. And the best thing, the ingredients are so much better than any store-bought alternative.

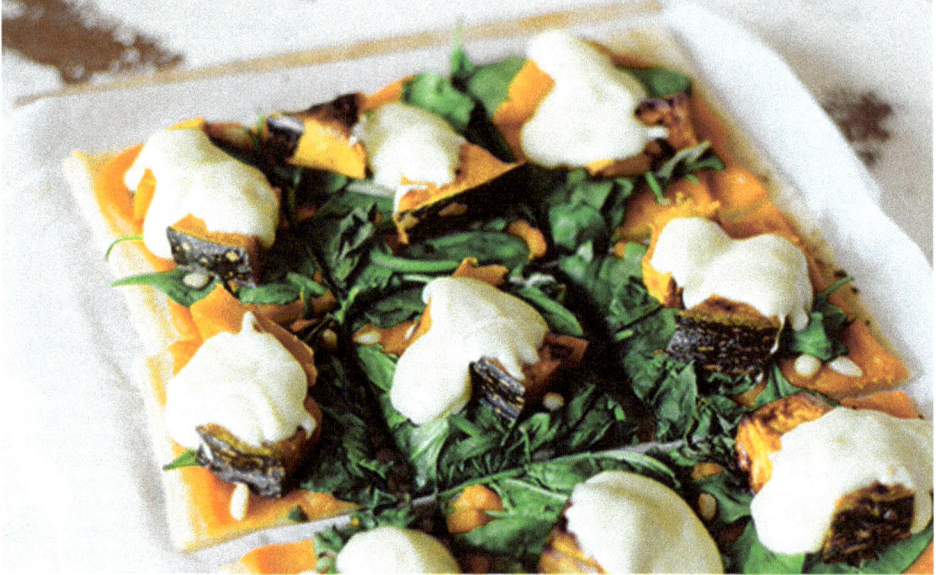

What's inside

- 1 cup water
- ¼ cup (35g) cashews, soaked and drained
- 2 ½ Tbs tapioca flour
- ½ garlic clove
- 1 Tbs of nutritional yeast
- 1 Tbs lemon juice (¼ a lemon)
- 1 tsp oregano
- ½ tsp sea salt

How to

1. Add all the ingredients to your blender and blend until you get a smooth texture. This will take about 2-3 minutes.
2. Pour the mixture into a small saucepan and heat over medium heat. Stir constantly to avoid any clumps. The texture will firm up after a couple of minutes.
3. The best way to enjoy the melting effect of this cheese is to immediately spoon it onto your pizza and enjoy straightaway. As it gets colder the cheese firms up.

Soft Cheddar

🕐 20 mins ⧗ 1 hr 🍴 1

The secret ingredients to this soft cheese is the miso – a paste made from fermented soy beans. Who would've thought that miso works well in dairy-free cheeze? Actually I'd say it's a taste wonder.

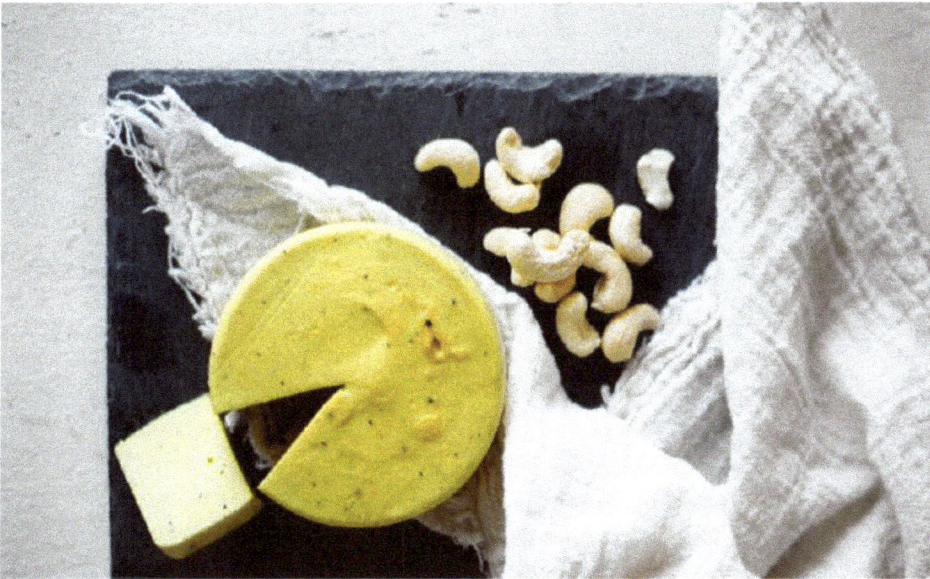

What's inside

- 1 ½ tsp agar agar powder
- ½ cup + ½ cup water
- ⅓ cup cashews, soaked and drained
- 1 Tbs + 2 tsp nutritional yeast
- 1 clove garlic, chopped
- 1 Tbs miso

- 1 ½ tsp arrowroot flour (or tapioca flour)
- 1 tsp turmeric
- 1 tsp sweet paprika
- 2 Tbs lemon juice (½ a lemon)
- ¼ tsp sea salt (optional)

How to

1. Add agar agar powder and ½ cup of water into a small saucepan, whisk and set aside.
2. Add all the ingredients to your blender and blend until you get a smooth texture. This will take about 2-3 minutes.

3. Pour the mix into the saucepan with the agar agar, and combine. Heat the pan to medium heat and stir constantly. At one point the mixture will suddenly thicken up (after about 3-5 minutes). Keep stirring to avoid clumps for about another 2-3 minutes.
4. Transfer the cheesy mix to a container and put it in the fridge until firm (at least 1 hour).

Nozzarella

🕐 15 mins   ⏳ 1 hr   🍴 15 cm roll

This nozzarella is a stunner on every brunch buffet. Just make sure you mention it's dairy-free, one of my friends didn't try it because he's lactose intolerant.

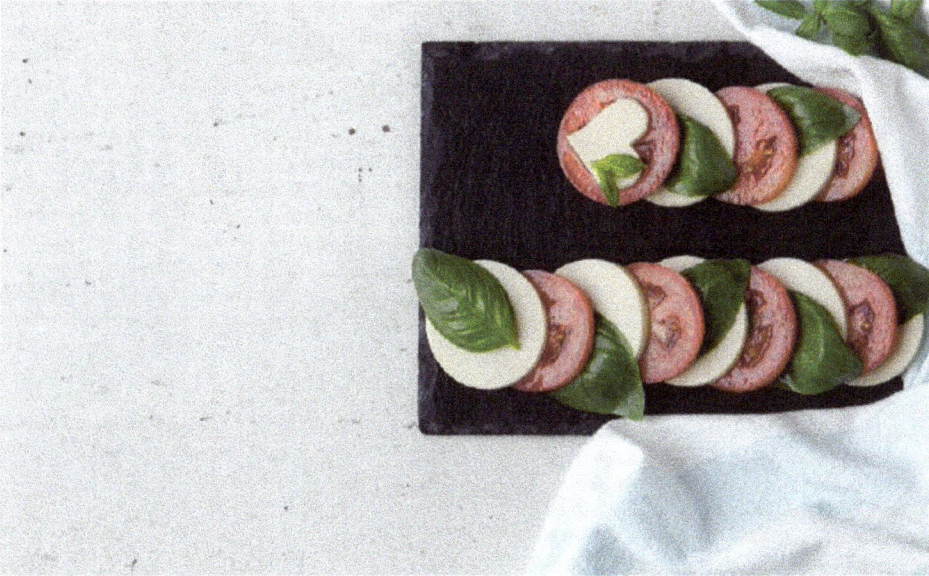

What's inside

- 1 ½ tsp agar agar powder
- ½ cup + ½ cup water
- ⅓ cup cashews, soaked and drained
- 1 Tbs + 2 tsp nutritional yeast
- 1 clove garlic
- 1 tsp mustard
- 1 ½ tsp arrowroot flour (or tapioca flour)
- 2 Tbs lemon juice (½ a lemon)
- ¼ tsp onion powder
- ¼ tsp sea salt

How to

1. Add agar agar powder and ½ cup of water into a small sauce pan, whisk and set aside.
2. Add all the ingredients to your blender and blend until you get a smooth texture. This will take about 2-3 minutes.
3. Pour the mix into the saucepan with the agar agar, and combine. Heat the pan to medium heat and stir constantly. At one point the mixture will

suddenly thicken up (after about 3-5 minutes). Keep stirring to avoid clumps for about another 2-3 minutes.

4. Transfer the cheesy mix to a container and put it in the fridge until firm (at least 1 hour).

Kitchen hack

- You will get 'real' looking mozzarella if you use a cut-open sauce tube to cool the mozzarella as it has the traditional round form.

Cheezy Nacho Sauce

🕐 10 mins ⏳ 0 mins 🍴 2

Oh wow – never miss this gooey cheesy nacho sauce again. The best thing about this version? It is actually moderately low in fat and high in protein. Plus it is sooo yum.

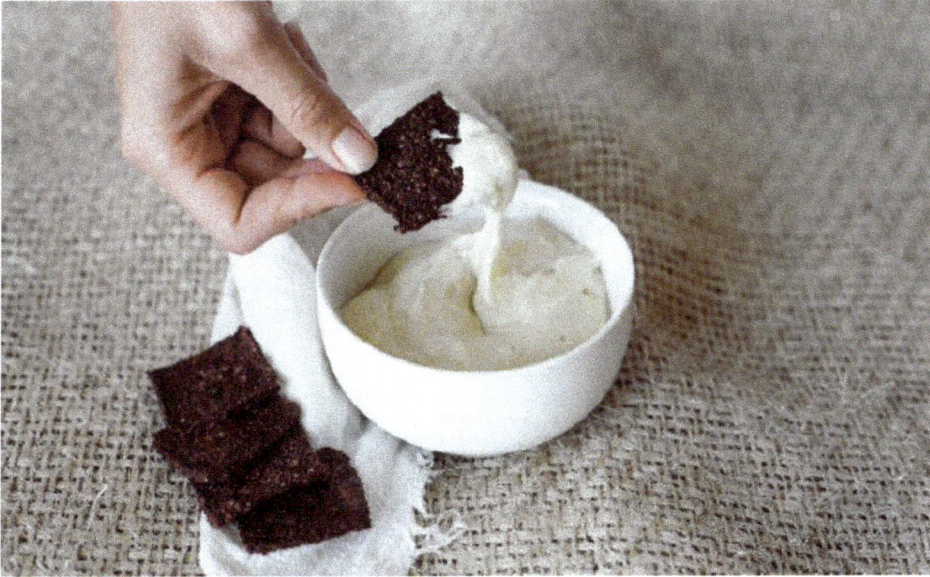

What's inside

- 100g tofu
- 2 Tbs corn flour
- 2 Tbs nutritional yeast
- ½ red onion
- 1 garlic cloves
- 1 cup water
- ½ tsp salt

How to

1. Add all the ingredients to your blender and blend until you get a really smooth texture. This will take about 2-3 minutes.
2. Pour the mix into a saucepan and heat to medium heat. Stir constantly. At one point the mixture will suddenly thicken up (after about 3-5 minutes). Keep stirring to avoid clumps for about another 2-3 minutes.
3. Transfer the cheesy mix to a bowl and dip your nachos in it. Enjoy hot or cold, however you prefer.

Swaps

- You can replace the tofu with 1 cup raw, soaked and drained cashew nuts.
- You can replace the corn flour with chickpea flour.
- You can replace the red onion with 3 spring onions.

Ultimate dairy-free Queso with Chili & Nachos

🕐 25 mins ⏳ 0 mins 🍴 2

The entertainer. The Queso & Chili Nachos are such a great meal to share with your friends and the queso has been tasted by hard-core Mexican food fans.

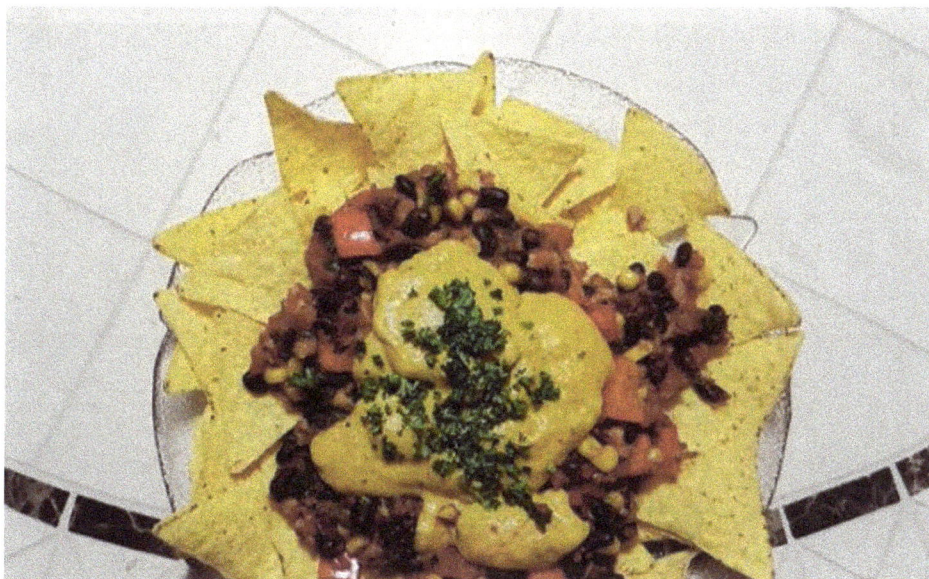

What's inside

- 1 bag of gluten-free corn nachos

Chili

- ½ onion, diced
- 1 corn, cut off the kernels
- 1/2 red capsicum
- 1 can black beans
- 1 can kidney or butter beans

- 1 can diced tomatoes
- 1 red chili
- Pepper to taste
- 2 Tbs fresh parsley

Queso

- 1 cup water
- 1/4 cup cashews, soaked and drained
- 2.5 Tbs arrowroot or tapioca flour
- 2 garlic cloves
- 1 tsp lemon juice

- 2 Tbs nutritional yeast
- 1 pinch turmeric
- 1/4 tsp onion powder
- 1/4 tsp hot paprika
- 1/4 tsp sweet paprika
- 1 pinch dried jalapeños

Hot Tofu Crunch (optional)
- 100g tofu
- 1 Tbs chilli flakes
- 1 tsp each paprika + pepper
- ½ tsp each cumin + coriander

How to

1. **Chili:** Add the onions to a medium sized saucepan and cook with 1/4 cup water until nice and soft.

2. Add the other ingredients, cook for about 5 minutes on medium heat until you get the desired consistency and temperature. Season to taste.

3. **Hot Tofu Crunch:** In a bowl, crush the tofu with a fork until it's broken into small crumbly pieces. Add the spices and mix until well combined. Heat a non-stick pan and add the tofu. Fry until it has a slightly golden colour. Stir regularly to avoid burning, this will take about 5-8 minutes. You can either stir the tofu directly through the chili or put it on top, once you plate up.

4. **Queso:** Add all ingredients to a blender and blend until everything is a smooth sauce (2-3 minutes). Pour the cheezy sauce into a cold saucepan and heat to medium heat. Stir constantly until the queso thickens which will take about 5 minutes.

5. **Plating-up:** Now it's time to plate everything up. First spread the nachos out on a large serving plate. Place them towards the sides of the plate, leaving the middle free. Pour the chili in the middle and try not to add too much on top of the nachos, as this makes them soggy and harder to eat. Next add the crunchy tofu on top of the chili. Finally, pour the queso on top and decorate with some fresh parsley, spring onions or jalapeño slices if you like. I also love it with some guacamole on the side.

Golden Sweet Potato Pumpkin Pizza

🕐 50 mins   ⧗ 0 mins   🍽 2

This pizza has been inspired by the I Quit Sugar 8 week program. It blew my mind! It is so flavoursome and incredibly smooth – and seriously, just look at those colours! It was my favourite recipe from the whole program and this cheeze is the perfect match.

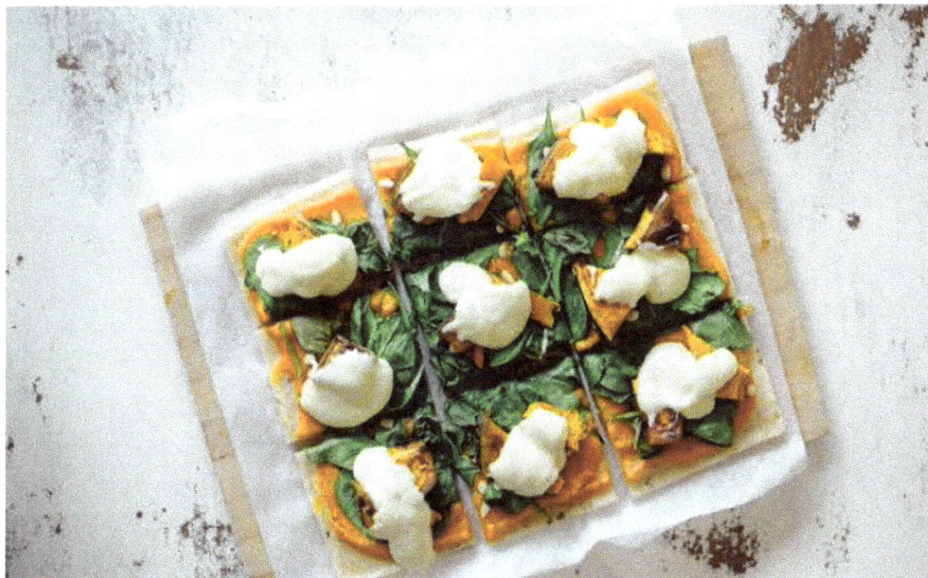

What's inside

- 2 gluten-free wraps or pizza base
- 1 big sweet potato, washed and quartered (200g)
- 1 small Kensington pumpkin, washed and quartered (400g)

- 2 Tbs rosemary
- 1 tsp pepper
- 2 Tbs pine nuts
- 2 cups spinach
- 1 handful basil leaves

Melting Pizza Cheeze
- 1 cup water
- ¼ cup cashews, soaked and drained
- 2 ½ Tbs tapioca flour
- ½ garlic clove

- 1 Tbs of nutritional yeast
- 1 Tbs lemon juice (¼ a lemon)
- 1 tsp oregano
- ½ tsp sea salt

How to
1. Preheat the oven to 180 degrees.

2. Add the sweet potato and pumpkin on a baking tray lined with parchment paper. Bake for about 20 minutes until soft and tender.

3. Add 2/3 of the sweet potato and pumpkin to a blender together with the rosemary and pepper and blend until well combined. Slice the remaining sweet potato & pumpkin.

4. Roast the pine nuts in a hot, dry pan for a couple of minutes. Make sure you don't burn them.

5. Put the pizza base on a baking tray covered with parchment paper. Spread the pumpkin-potato sauce on top. Add the basil & spinach leaves and top it with the sliced veggies & roasted pine nuts. Cook for another 15 minutes until the greens are soft.

6. Meanwhile, to make the melting pizza cheese, add all the ingredients to your blender and blend until you get a smooth, fine texture. This will take about 2-3 minutes.

7. Pour the mixture into a small saucepan and heat over medium heat. Stir constantly to avoid any clumps. The texture will firm up after a couple of minutes.

8. The best way to enjoy the melting effect of this cheese is to immediately spoon it onto your pizza and enjoy straightaway. As it gets colder the cheese firms up.

9. Take the pizza out of the oven and spoon the melting pizza cheese just before serving!

Kitchen hack

- I like to cook a big batch of sweet potato pumpkin puree and freeze the leftover for the next time I make this pizza. This reduces the cook time significantly and I can have it as a super quick dinner pizza.

Pear & Walnut Salad with Crumbly Macadamia Cheeze

🕐 15 mins ⏳ 0 mins 🍴 2

One of my favourite salads. Super quick, packed with nutrients, yes even heaps of omega 3, naturally sweetened with pears and rich, thanks to the crumbly cheeze and walnuts.

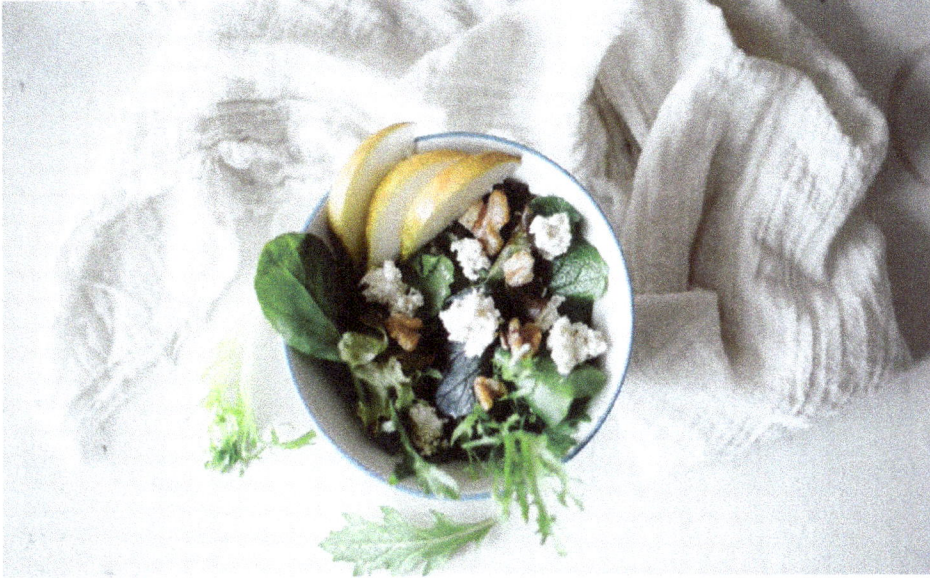

What's inside
- 3 handfuls of rocket
- 1 handful of basil leaves
- 1 pear, finely sliced
- ¼ cup walnuts, crushed
- ¼ cup crumbly macadamia cheeze

Dressing
- 1 Tbs Dijon mustard
- 1 Tbs apple cider vinegar
- 1 dash cinnamon and turmeric
- pepper to taste

How to
1. Mix all ingredients for the dressing.
2. Add rocket and basil to a salad bowl and fold under the dressing.
3. Divide between two plates and decorate with pear, walnuts and cheese.

Kitchen hack
- As it is easier in most food processors to do a larger batch of the crumbly cheese, I've included the recipe for ½ cup. Simply store the left-over in an airtight container in the fridge and enjoy later.

SPREADS & DIPS

Quick German Spelt Bread

🕐 10 mins   ⧗ 45 mins   🍴 1 large loaf

This bread is not only super quick and delicious, it is also German taste test approved. It was my lifesaver when I first moved to Australia as I was missing my good old German bread so badly.

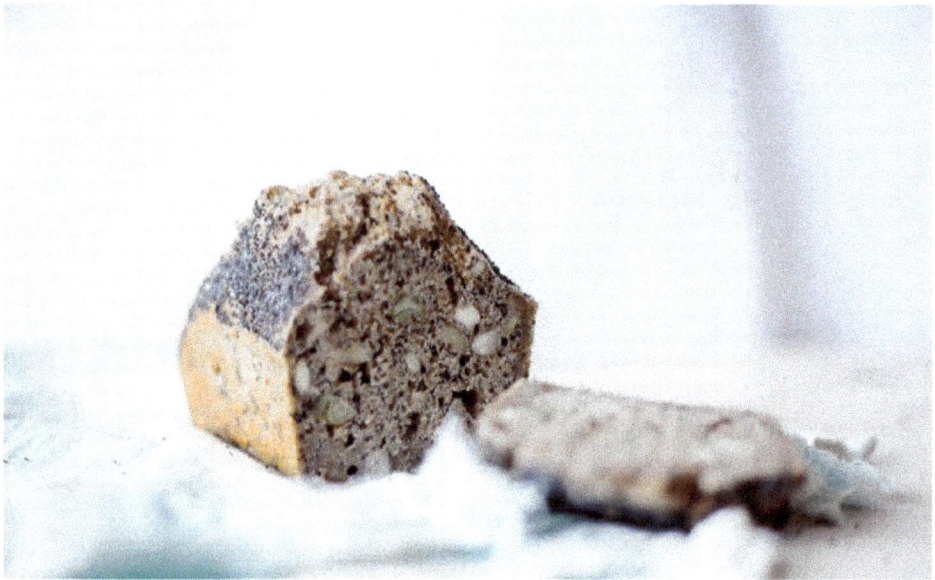

What's inside
- 500g spelt flour
- 150g mixed seeds (poppy, sesame, pepitas, sunflower)
- 4g dry yeast
- 2 cups water

How to
1. Line a loaf tin with baking paper.
2. Preheat the oven to 250°C.
3. Add all the ingredients in the order above to a mixing bowl. Mix well immediately.
4. Pour the dough into a loaf tin and put it directly into the oven on the middle tray for 30 – 45 minutes.

5. After 10 minutes, cut the top of the bread with a sharp knife to avoid uncontrolled cracking.
6. Once the bread is ready you will smell it. Test it by sticking a toothpick into the bread. If it comes out clean, it's ready; if there is still some dough on it, leave it in for another 2-3 minutes before you test again. You can also switch off the oven at this point, the remaining heat will be enough.

Superpower Seed Bread (gluten-free)

🕐 15 mins ⏳ 0 mins 🍽 2

Being German I do love my bread and this one is incredible. Yes, it does take some time to bake and let me tell you it is absolutely worth it. A couple of restaurant owners already asked me if I'd produce it for them. You can bake a bigger loaf, slice it up and freeze it until you feel like a piece of bread.

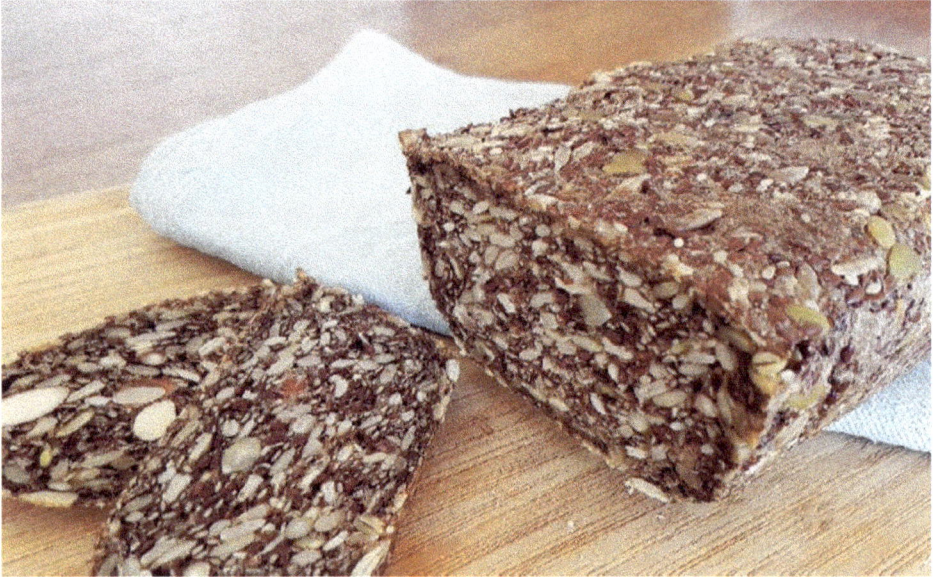

What's inside

- 1 ½ cups sunflower seeds
- ¾ cup pepitas
- ½ cup buckwheat
- ½ cup almonds
- ¾ cup flaxseeds
- 1 Tbs sesame seeds
- 2 Tbs chia seeds
- 4 Tbs psyllium husk
- 1 tsp sea salt
- 1 ½ cup water
- 1 tsp slippery elm

How to

1. Line a loaf tin with baking paper.
2. Add all the ingredients to a bowl and combine well.
3. Pour the bread mix into the loaf tin and let stand for 2 hours.
4. After 1 hour and 45 minutes, preheat the oven to 175°C.

5. Put the loaf on the middle tray and bake for about 1 hour until the top of the loaf is crisp.
6. Take the bread out of the oven and immediately close the door again. Turn off the oven.
7. Remove the bread from the tin and baking paper. Put it upside down back on the baking rack and return it to the oven with the remaining heat for another hour. You can test if it's done by knocking on it; if it sounds hollow, it's ready.

Cashew Cream Cheese

🕐 15 mins   ⧗ 0 mins   🍴 1.5 cups

Even though this cream cheese is not as good as the one from Peace Love and Vegetables, it is a lot cheaper and you can make as much as you actually need and on demand. Plus a kitchen creative like me can play with the ingredients and add all kinds of herbs. Oh and you can fill zucchini flowers with it – THE best dairy-free dish ever. It looks like it's made by a trained chef and is seriously so much fun to make. Simply fill the flowers, bake for 10–15 minutes and enjoy the little beauty.

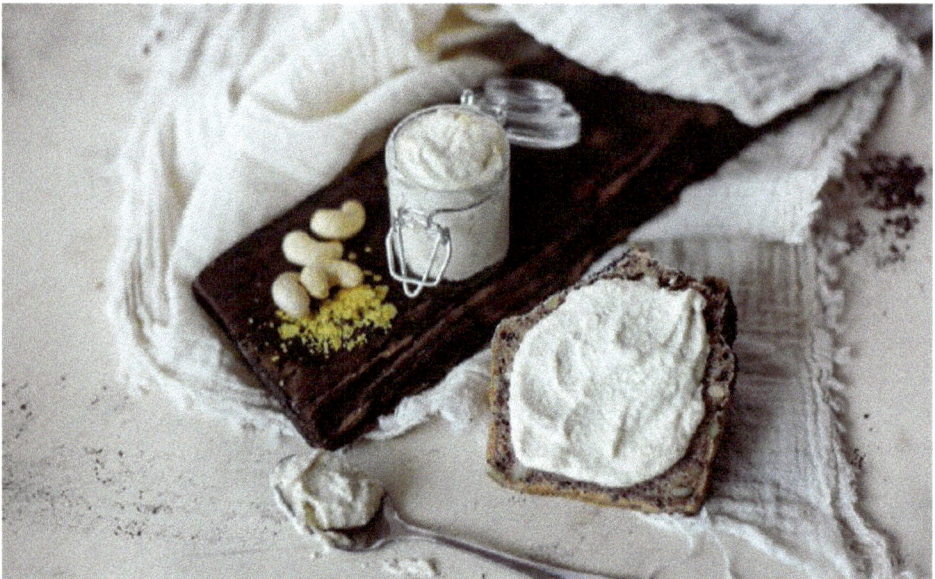

What's inside

- 1 cup cashews, soaked and drained
- ¼ cup water
- 2 Tbs lemon juice (half a lemon)
- 1 garlic clove
- 1 Tbs nutritional yeast
- 1 tsp dried rosemary
- 1 tsp dried oregano

How to

1. Add all the ingredients to your blender and blend.
2. Occasionally turn the blender off and scrape down the cheese until you get a smooth texture. This will take about 2-3 minutes.
3. Adjust the consistency by adding more or less water. Play around a bit until you get your preferred consistency.

Newtella

🕐 5 mins   ⧗ 0 mins   🍽 1/2 cup

All my life I have been a massive Nutella addict. My mother in law once said, 'What if Nutella is causing you headaches – have you tried not having it?' I told her I'd rather have headaches than give up my Nutella. Fast forward – 2 years ago I made a blind tasting and hands down, this Newtella was my absolute favourite. It's not only dairy-free and delicious, the ingredients are next level.

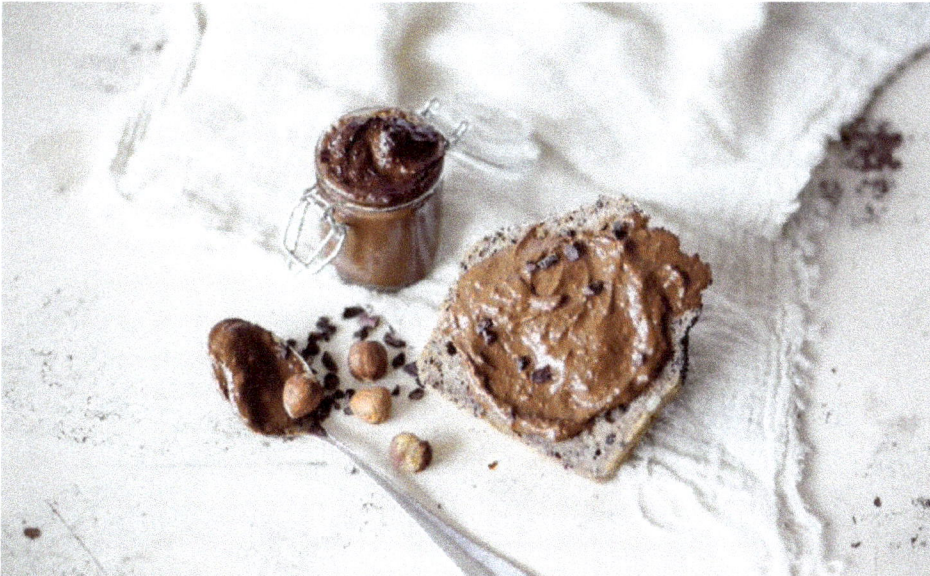

What's inside

- ⅓ cup hazelnut butter
- 2 Tbs cacao
- 2 Tbs coconut sugar
- 4 Tbs coconut cream
- 1 tsp vanilla (optional)

How to

1. Add all the ingredients to a bowl and mix until everything is well combined.

Kitchen hack

- Be careful if you mix it in a food processor; be sure to avoid overheating as this can give your newtella a sticky consistency.
- If you prefer a smoother consistency which gets firmer when chilled, simply add some coconut oil (about 1 tablespoon).

Swap

- For an oil-free version: Swap the coconut cream for your favourite mylk, like hazelnut mylk.
- For a cheaper alternative use ¼ cup raw, soaked cashews or almonds and add 1-2 tablespoons hazelnuts for the taste.

Best Peanut Butter

🕐 5 mins   ⧗ 0 mins   🍴 3 cups

#kidsapproved. One day a friend of mine went sugar-free with her family, which meant their favourite peanut butter was off the menu. Her kids started a peanut butter rebellion. As a peanut butter addict I totally got that and went straight to the drawing board—aka my pantry—to recreate a this healthy version of sweet peanut butter.

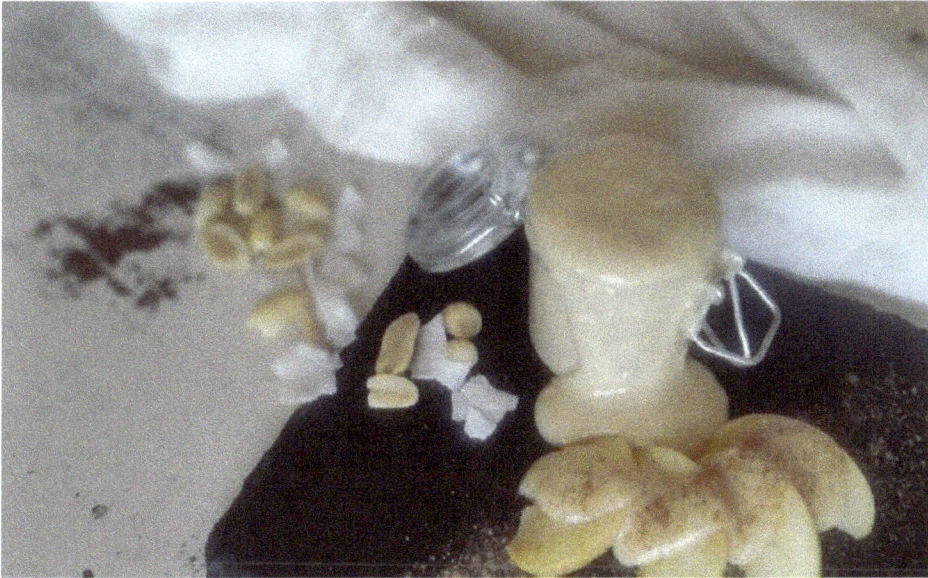

What's inside
- 2 cups peanuts
- 1 cup coconut flakes

How to
1. Put the peanuts and coconut flakes in a blender and blend.
2. Occasionally turn the blender off and scrape down the peanut butter until you get a smooth texture.

Variation
- Experiment with cinnamon or vanilla as well as cacao nibs.

Hot Spread

🕐 15 mins   ⏳ 0 mins   🍴 1 ½ cups

In Germany we eat a lot of bread and I do like a nice sandwich for lunch. So there was the question of "what can you spread on it when cream cheese is off the menu?" This hot spread is delicious and a man's favourite :)

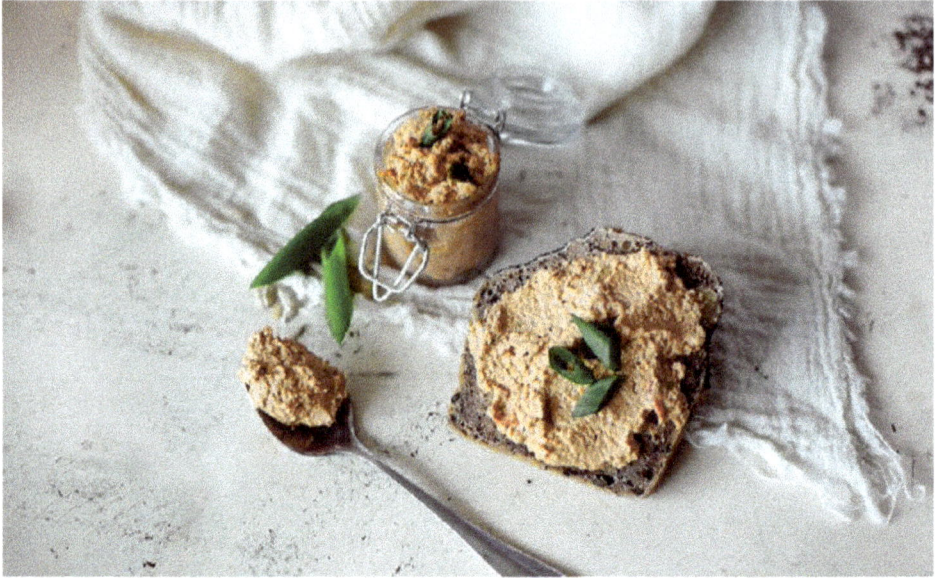

What's inside

- ½ cup sunflower seeds, soaked and drained
- ¼ cup water
- ½ cup tomato paste
- ¼ brown onion
- 1 garlic clove
- 1 Tbs lemon juice (¼ a lemon)
- 1 tsp paprika hot
- 1 Tbs paprika mild
- ½ tsp chilli powder (or ½ a small chilli)
- 1 tsp pepper
- salt to taste (optional)

How to

1. Add all the ingredients to your blender and blend.
2. Occasionally turn the blender off and scrape down the spread until you get a smooth texture. This will take about 3-5 minutes.
3. Adjust the consistency by adding more or less water. Play around a bit until you get your preferred consistency.

Swap

- If you prefer a firmer, oilier consistency you can substitute some water with sunflower oil.

Tomato Spread

🕐 15 mins ⏳ 0 mins 🍴 1 ½ cups

The softer version of our nut-free bread spreads. A couple of years back I actually planned to produce these spreads commercially. Plans changed and now you get the recipe. So enjoy!

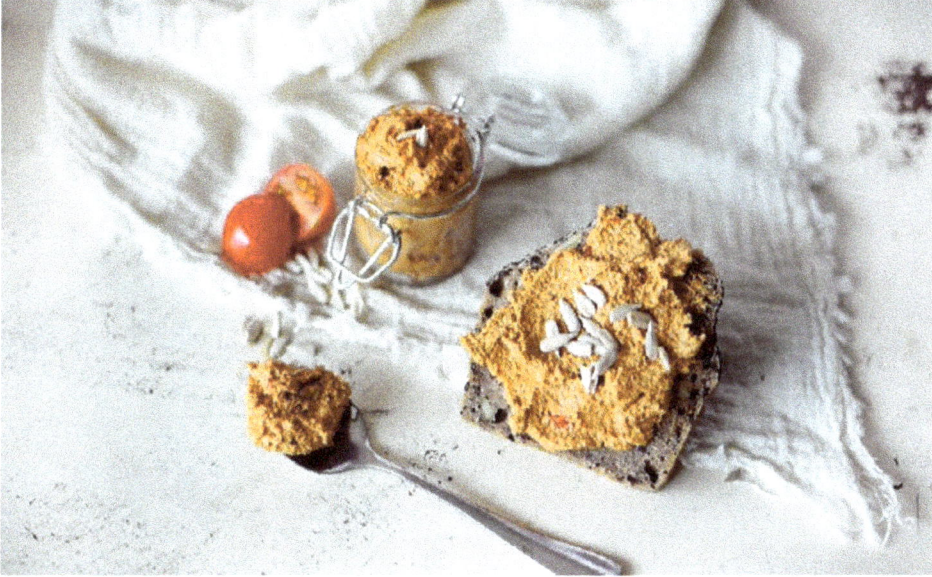

What's inside

- ½ cup sunflower seeds, soaked and drained
- ¼ cup water
- ½ cup tomato paste
- ¼ brown onion
- 1 Tbs lemon juice (¼ a lemon)
- 1 Tbs oregano dried
- 1 tsp pepper

How to

1. Add all the ingredients to your blender and blend.
2. Occasionally turn the blender off and scrape down the spread until you get a smooth texture. This will take about 3-5 minutes.
3. Adjust the consistency by adding more or less water. Play around a bit until you get your preferred consistency.

Swap

- If you prefer a firmer, oilier consistency you can substitute some water with sunflower oil.

Hummus

🕐 10 mins   ⧗ 0 mins   🍴 1 1/2 cups

My go-to snack. It's amazing with veggies and really fills you up. I sometimes have a small jar for lunch.

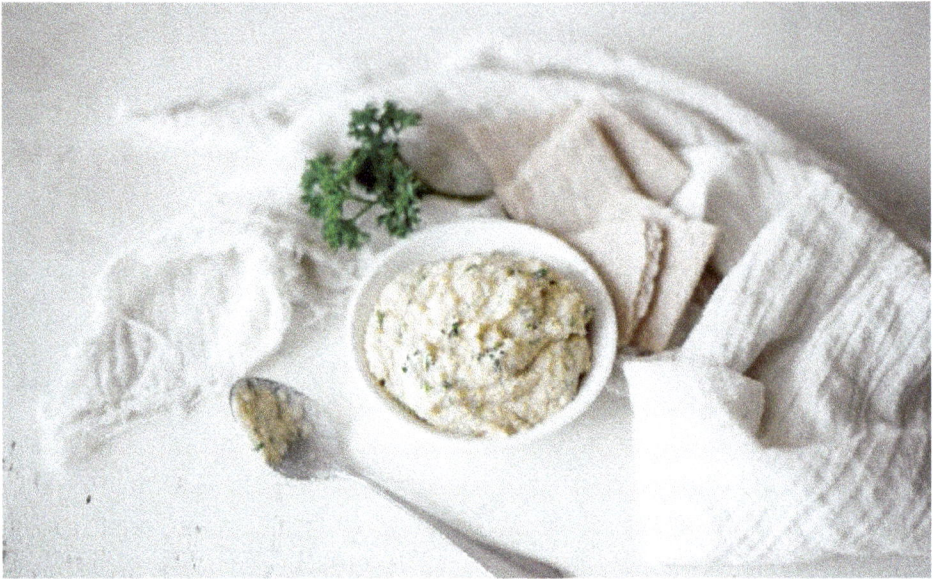

What's inside

- 1 can chickpeas, drained
- 2 Tbs tahini
- 2 Tbs lemon juice (½ a lemon)
- ½ cup water
- 1 garlic clove
- 1 Tbs pepper
- Fresh parsley

How to

1. Add all the ingredients except the parsley to your blender and blend.
2. Occasionally turn the blender off and scrap down the hummus until you get a smooth texture. This will take about 2-3 minutes.
3. Adjust the consistency by adding more or less water. Play around a bit until you get your preferred consistency.
4. Lastly, stir through the parsley.

Guacamole

🕐 10 mins ⧗ 0 mins 🍴 1/2 cup

In our house guacamole is a food staple. We have it at least once a week, with corn chips, veggies, on burgers or even as a dip with pizza and if we're really sneaky I might just have it by itself. Cannot resist its creaminess…

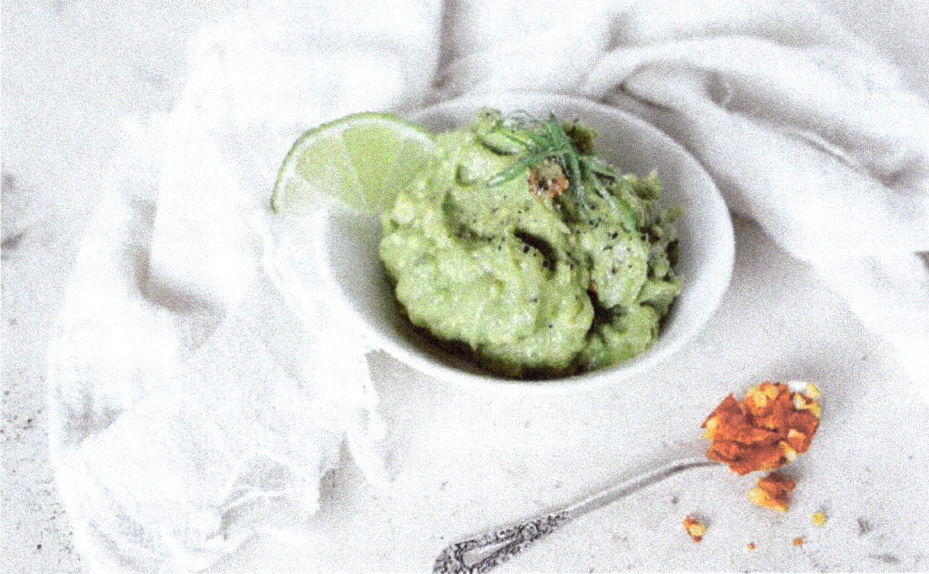

What's inside

- 1 avocado
- ½ a lime, juiced
- 1 small chilli, finely cut
- 1 garlic clove, finely cut
- ½ a spring onion, thinly cut
- 1 handful coriander, roughly cut

How to

1. Mash the avocado with a fork.
2. Use a pestle and mortar to grind the garlic and chilli.
3. Place all the ingredients in a bowl and combine well.

Beetroot Almond Dip

🕐 10 mins ⏳ 0 mins 🍴 1/2 cup

Look at those colours – This dip is the perfect companion for any starter. It's smooth, flavoursome and soooo good. Nobody would guess it's dairy-free.

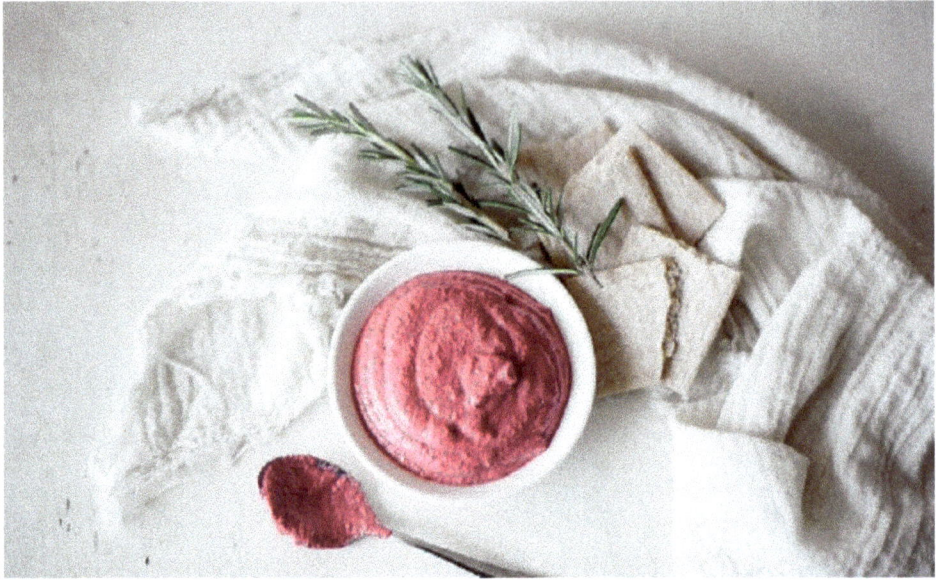

What's inside

- 2 cooked medium-sized beetroots
- 4 Tbs almond butter
- 1 tsp Dijon mustard
- 4 Tbs water
- 2 tsp fresh rosemary
- ½ tsp pepper

How to

1. Add all the ingredients to your blender and blend.
2. Occasionally turn the blender off and scrape down the dip until you get a smooth texture. This will take about 2-3 minutes.
3. Adjust the consistency by adding more or less water. Play around a bit until you get your preferred consistency.

Sour Cream

🕐 10 mins   ⧗ 0 mins   🍴 1 1/2 cup

As a child I would cook lunch every Friday for my mum and sister. I loved it – I guess that's when my passion for cooking was born. One of our favourites dishes was baked potatoes with sour cream – simple yet delicious. Here is my dairy-free take on sour cream.

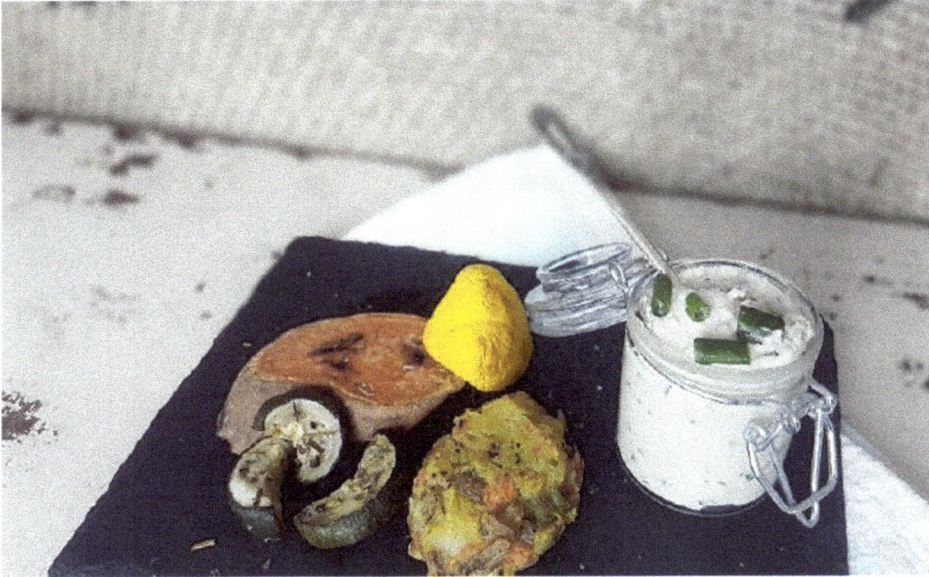

What's inside

- ⅓ cup water
- 1 cup raw cashews, soaked and drained
- 2 Tbs lemon juice (½ a lemon)
- 2 tsp apple cider vinegar
- 1 Tbs nutritional yeast
- ½ bunch chives, chopped

How to

1. Add all the ingredients except the chives to your blender and blend.
2. Occasionally turn the blender off and scrape down the mixture until you get a smooth texture. This will take about 2-3 minutes.
3. Check the taste and add more lemon juice for a tangier taste, or more water for a runnier consistency.
4. Transfer the sour cream into a bowl and fold in the chives.

PASTA SAUCES

2 Ingredient Cooking Cream

🕐 5 mins   ⧗ 0 mins   🍴 1 cup

This 2 ingredient cooking cream is a true life changer – never think about buying cooking cream again, all you need are cashews and water. There are no leftovers that can go off and there are no nasties inside.

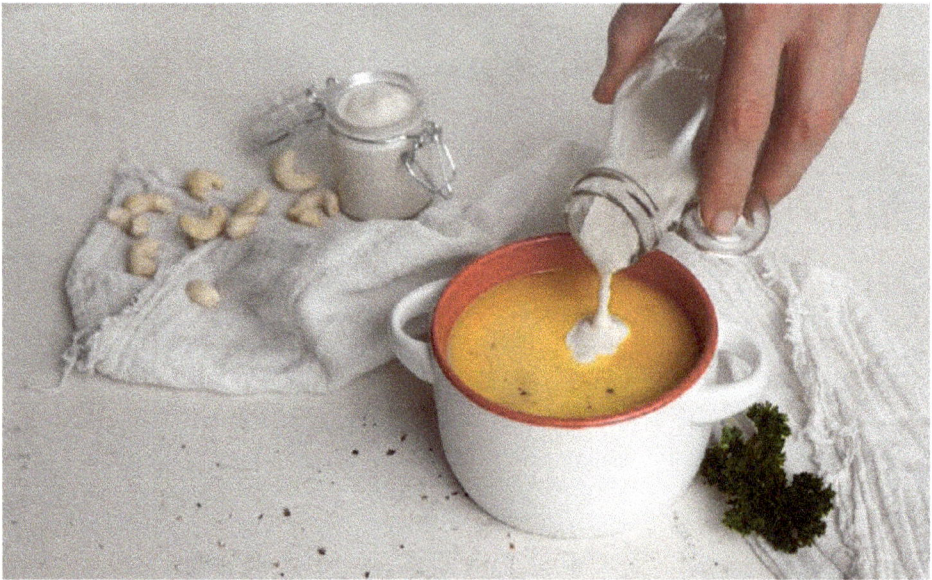

What's inside
- ½ cup water
- ½ cup raw cashews, soaked and drained

How to
1. Add all the ingredients to your blender and blend.
2. Occasionally turn the blender off and scrape down the cream until you get a smooth texture. This will take about 2 minutes (depending on your blender).

Kitchen hack
- If you plan to blend the sauce or soup you're cooking, you can simply add the nuts and water together with sauce / soup and blend everything together. There's no need to pre-blend the cooking cream.

Creamy Capsicum Pasta

🕐 10 mins   ⧗ 0 mins   🍴 2

Long day at work? No time for cooking? This recipe is for you. It's my absolute favourite summer dish, refreshing, wholesome and filled with pure goodness.

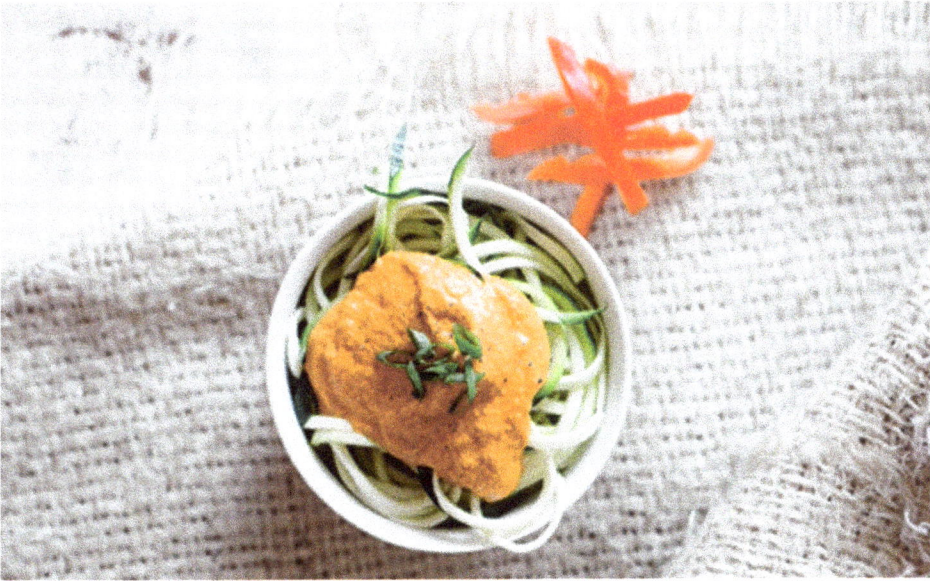

What's inside

- 4 zucchini
- 2 red capsicums
- 4 spring onions
- 2 garlic cloves
- 1 tsp sweet paprika
- ½ cup water
- ⅓ cup cashews, soaked and drained

How to

1. Use the thin blade of your spiralizer to make zucchini noodles. Keep the leftover for later.
2. Add all remaining ingredients plus the leftover zucchini to your blender and blend.
3. Occasionally turn the blender off and scrape down the sauce until you get a smooth texture. This will take about 1-2 minutes.
4. Optional: Pour the sauce into a saucepan and heat it up.
5. Add the zoodles (zucchini noodles) to the sauce, stir through and enjoy.

Kitchen hack

- If you cook the sauce, try not to let it boil (ideally keep the temperature below 50C), this way you will preserve the valuable minerals and nutrients.

Mac 'n' Cheese

🕐 20 mins   ⧗ 0 mins   🍴 2

My sister loves the US so of course I had to re-create this American classic into a delicious and nourishing alternative. Both the big and small kids will love it.

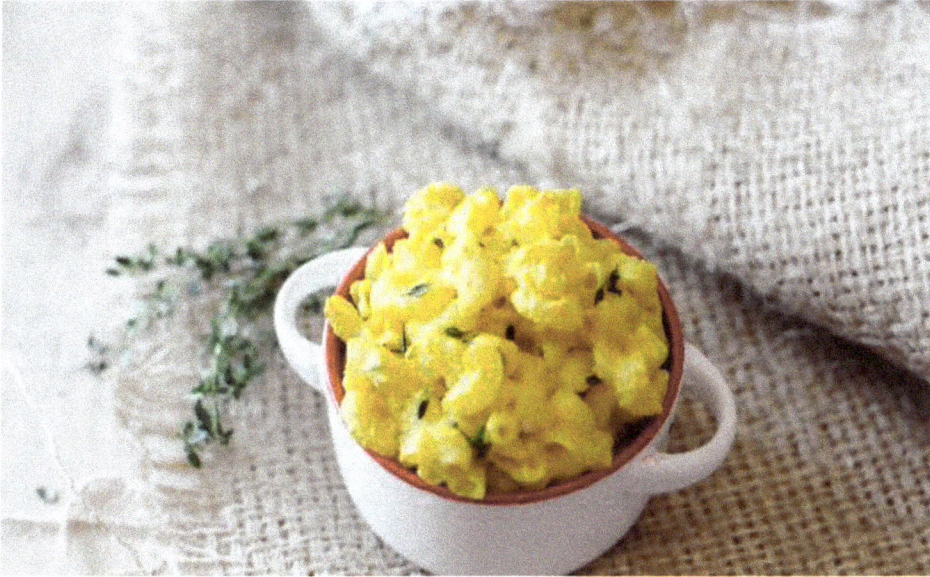

What's inside

- 200g mini macaroni
- 1 cup cashews, soaked and drained
- 1 garlic clove
- 1 small spring onion
- 3 Tbs nutritional yeast
- 2 tsp mustard
- 1 tsp turmeric
- ½ tsp sweet paprika
- 1 tsp thyme
- 1 cup water
- Salt and pepper to taste
- 2 Tbs 'nutty parmesan' (optional)

How to

1. Preheat your oven to 180°C degrees.
2. Cook the pasta.
3. Meanwhile, add all the ingredients except the pasta to your blender and blend.
4. Occasionally turn the blender off and scrape down the sauce until you get a smooth texture. This will take about 2-3 minutes.

5.   Drain the pasta and transfer into a large bowl. Add the sauce and mix until everything is well combined.

6.   Fill small ramekins with the pasta and sprinkle 'nutty parmesan' on top.

7.   Put the ramekins in the oven and bake for about 10 minutes.

Creamy Mushroom Pasta

🕐 15 mins ⏳ 0 mins 🍴 2

This is one of my favourite pasta dishes. It is hearty, creamy and deliciously rich in flavour. Make sure you use a good red wine though.

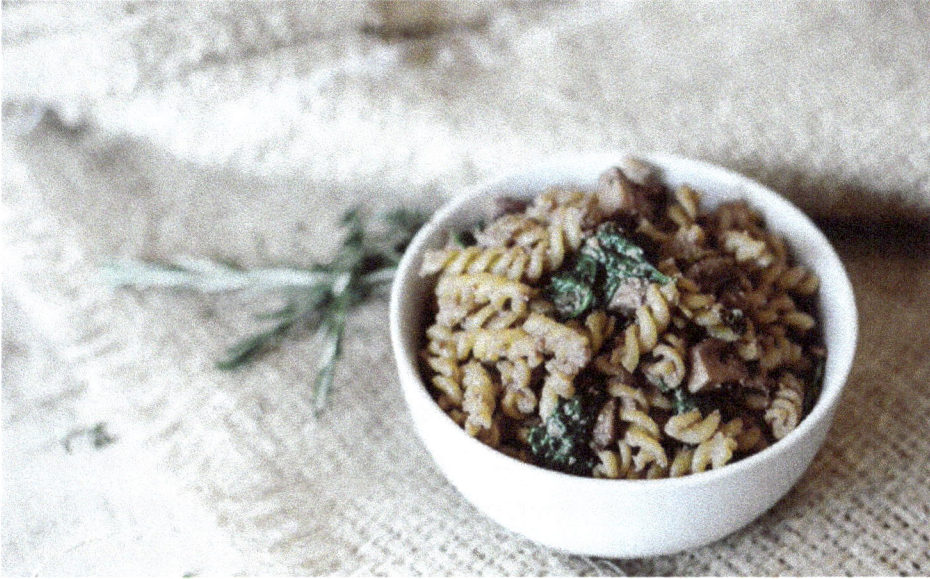

What's inside

- 250g pasta
- 1 Tbs tamari sauce
- 2 Tbs almond flour (or another gluten-free flour)
- 1 Tbs nutritional yeast
- 1 cup water
- 2 spring onions, finely chopped
- 1 garlic clove, finely chopped
- ¼ cup red wine
- 10 mushrooms, sliced
- 2 Tbs fresh rosemary, chopped
- 2 handfuls spinach

How to

1. Cook the pasta.
2. In a bowl, mix tamari sauce, almond flour, nutritional yeast and water. Set aside.
3. Add 3 tablespoons water to a non-stick pan and heat to a high-medium heat. Add the spring onions and garlic, cook for 1-2 minutes and then deglaze with the red wine.

4. Add the mushrooms and rosemary, and fry for another minute.
5. Pour the tamari-flour mix into the pan while continually stirring and add the spinach. Cook for 2 more minutes.
6. Drain the pasta and add it to the sauce. Combine the sauce and the pasta and decorate with some rosemary before serving.

Basil Pesto

🕐 10 mins   ⧗ 0 mins   🍽 1 cup

When I first travelled through Australia as a backpacker I had pasta with pesto and fresh cocktail tomatoes pretty much every day. Today pesto always reminds me of my amazing time back in 2008. This straightforward pesto is super yummy. Nobody will taste the difference.

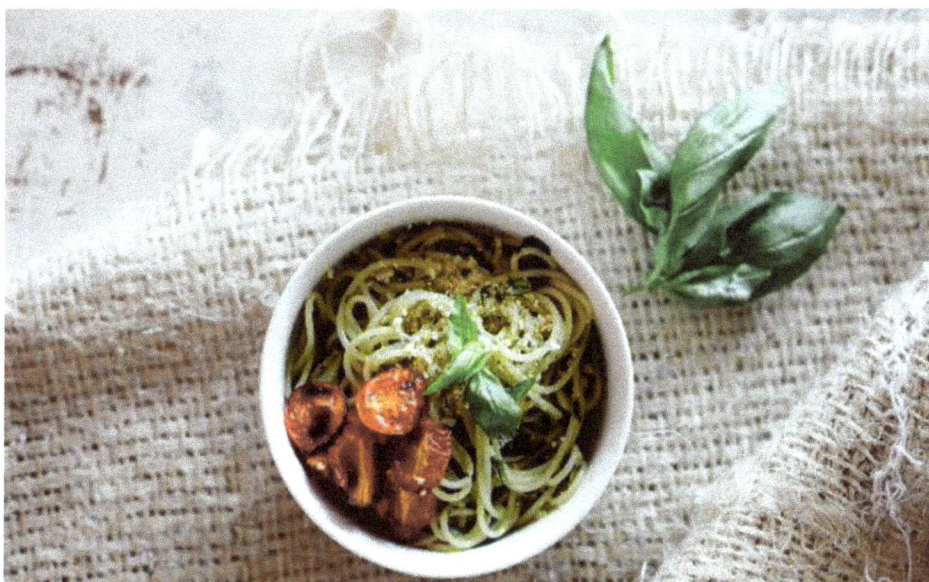

What's inside

- 1 bunch basil (2 handfuls)
- 1 garlic clove, diced
- ½ tsp salt
- 2 Tbs pine nuts (15g)
- 2 tsp nutritional yeast
- ½ cup olive oil
- Squeeze of lemon juice (optional)

How to

1. Pulse the basil, garlic and salt for a couple of seconds in your food processor.
2. Add the pine nuts and nutritional yeast, and pulse again until well combined.
3. While mixing, slowly add the olive oil and lemon juice.

Swap

- For an oil-free version: Skip the olive oil and add ½ an avocado to create a beautiful creamy texture.
- You can swap the pine nuts for other nuts like cashews or almonds.

Alfredo Sauce

🕐 20 mins   ⏳ 0 mins   🍽 2

Yuuuum – think of a soft creamy sauce that does not only work beautifully for pasta, you can turn it into a veggie bake; simply add heaps of veggies, mix it, bake it for a little bit and enjoy.

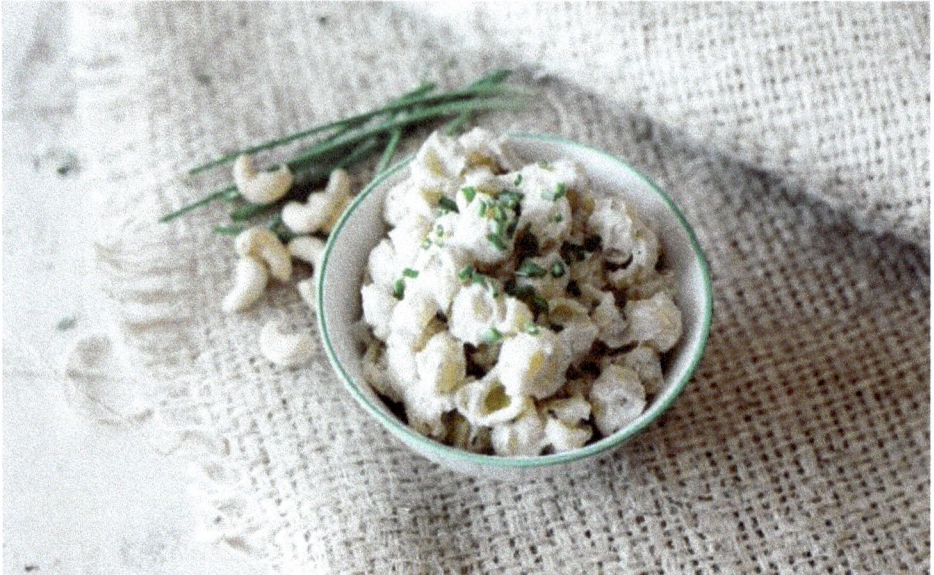

What's inside

- 250g pasta
- 3 small potatoes, cooked
- ½ a brown onion
- ⅓ cup cashews, soaked and drained
- 1 Tbs nutritional yeast
- ½ cup hot water
- 1 tsp freshly cracked pepper
- 1 pinch of nutmeg
- 1 cup frozen peas
- ½ bunch chives, roughly chopped

How to

1. Cook the pasta.
2. Meanwhile, add the potatoes, onion, cashews, nutritional yeast, water, pepper and nutmeg to your blender and blend.
3. Occasionally turn the blender off and scrape down the sauce until you get a smooth texture. This will take about 2-3 minutes.
4. Cover the frozen peas with hot water, and let them sit for 1-2 minutes before draining.

5. Pour the sauce into a bowl and stir through the peas and chives.
6. Add the cooked pasta to the sauce, stir through and decorate with the chives before serving.

Variation

- **Quick Pasta Bake:**
  In a baking dish, combine the pasta and sauce together with mixed blanched veggies like corn, capsicum, broccoli and carrots. Sprinkle some 'nutty parmesan' on top and bake at 200°C degrees for 10-15 minutes. Done and ready to enjoy.

Walnut Pesto

🕐 10 mins ⏳ 0 mins 🍴 1 cup

Such a beautiful variation of the traditional basil pesto. It works amazingly well with veggies and pasta as well.

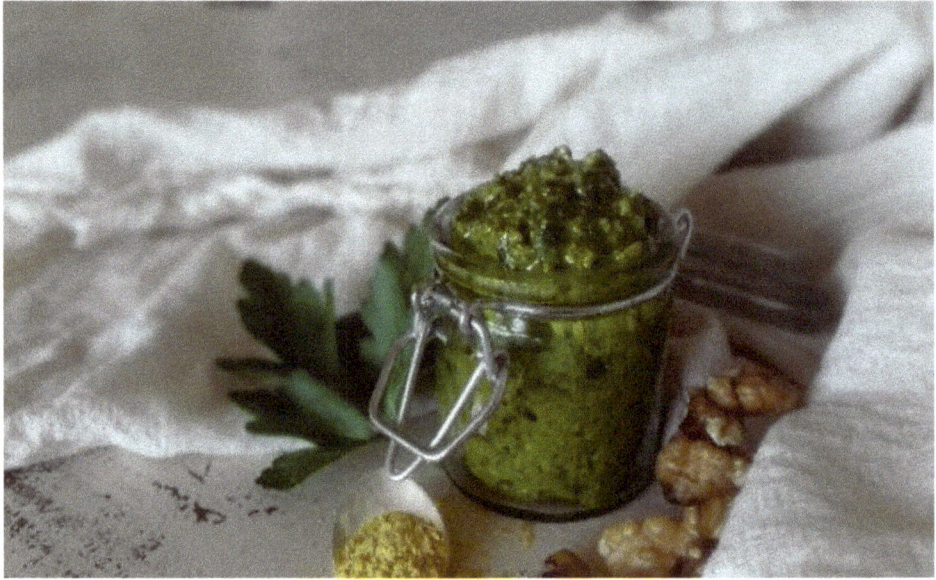

What's inside

- ½ bunch parsley (1 ½ cups)
- ⅓ cup walnuts
- 2 garlic cloves
- ¼ cup nutritional yeast
- ½ cup olive oil
- salt and pepper to taste

How to

1. Pulse the parsley, walnuts, garlic and nutritional yeast for a couple of seconds in your food processor.
2. While mixing, slowly add the olive oil until everything is well combined. Adjust the quantity of oil to your preference.
3. Season with salt and pepper to taste.

Swap

- For an oil-free version: Skip the olive oil and add ½ an avocado to create a beautiful creamy texture.

SWEET TREATS

Cacao Bliss Balls

🕐 10 mins   ⏳ 0 mins   🍴 12 balls

Sweet and yummy bliss balls without a ton of dates. Impossible? These Cacao Bliss Balls are the perfect travel companion, especially for long distance flights.

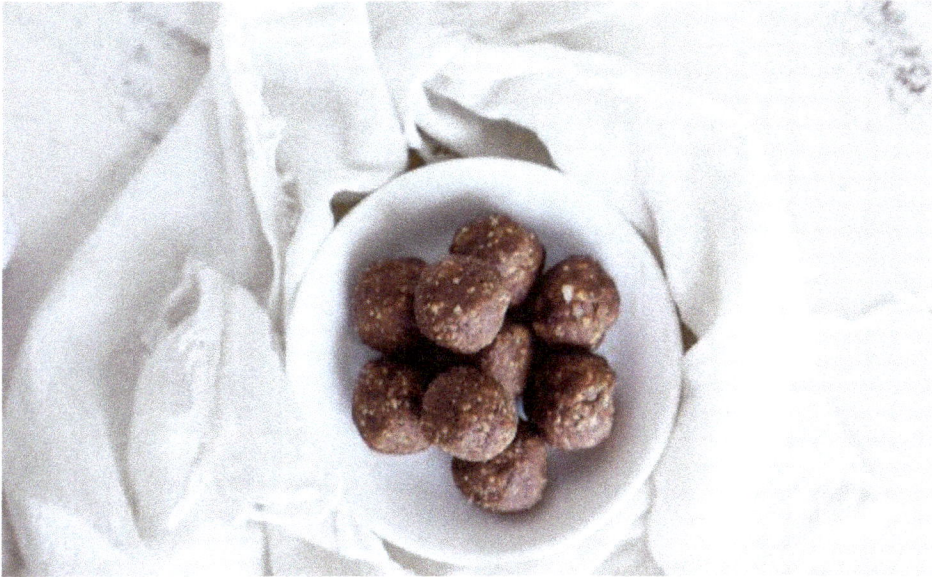

What's inside

- ½ cup smooth peanut butter
- 1 Tbs cacao
- 1 Tbs maple syrup
- ¼ cup dried banana
- ½ vanilla powder

How to

1. Blend all the ingredients until well combined.
2. Take out tablespoon-sized pieces and carefully press together to form balls with your hands.
3. Store in an airtight container in your fridge.

Kitchen hack

- If the dough is too dry and doesn't stick, add some additional peanut butter.

Swap

- You can swap the peanut butter for any other nut butter, like almond butter.

Coconut Bliss Balls

🕐 10 mins ⏳ 0 mins 🍽 12 balls

My dad and I are the biggest coconut macaroon fans on earth. Every year for Christmas we would make a big batch of them. The cool thing about these balls is the fact that I don't even have to wait for the oven any longer *hehe*

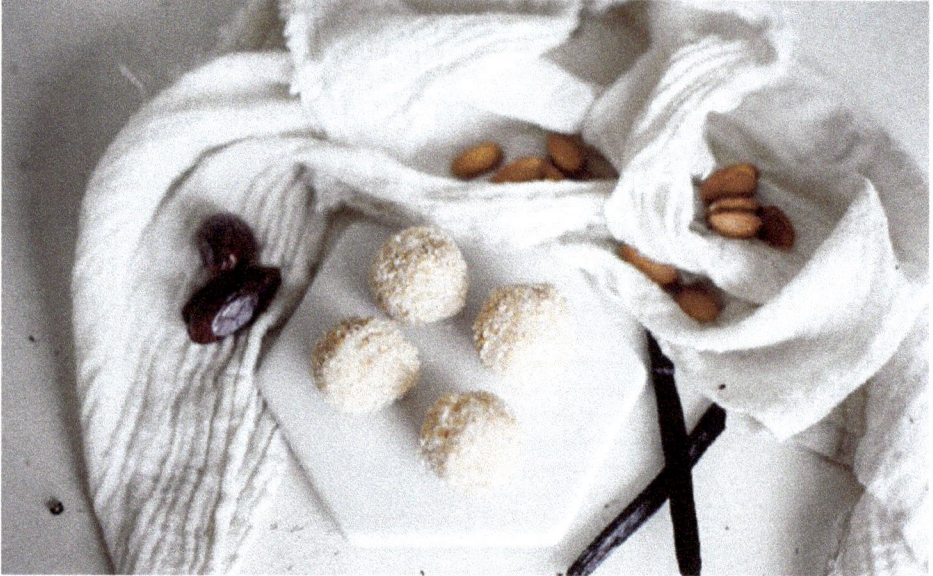

What's inside

- ½ cup unsweetened desiccated coconut flakes
- 1 date, soaked and drained
- 2 tsp almond butter
- 1 pinch vanilla powder

How to

1. Blend all the ingredients until well combined.
2. Take out tablespoon-sized pieces and carefully press together to form balls with your hands.
3. Store in an airtight container in your fridge.

Kitchen hack

- If the dough is too dry and doesn't stick, add some additional almond butter.
- For this beautiful white look your need to make your own almond butter. First soak the almonds, take off their skins and blend them in a high-speed blender until you get a smooth paste.

Mousse au Chocolate

🕐 5 mins   ⧖ 0 mins   🍴 1 cup

After trying the dairy-free lifestyle for 2 months, I re-tested my body's capability to digest dairy with a spoonful of mousse au chocolate at our favourite Italian place. I used the double dose lactaid and felt terribly ill within minutes. I went straight home and created this recipe. Gosh I cannot tell you how much I love it.

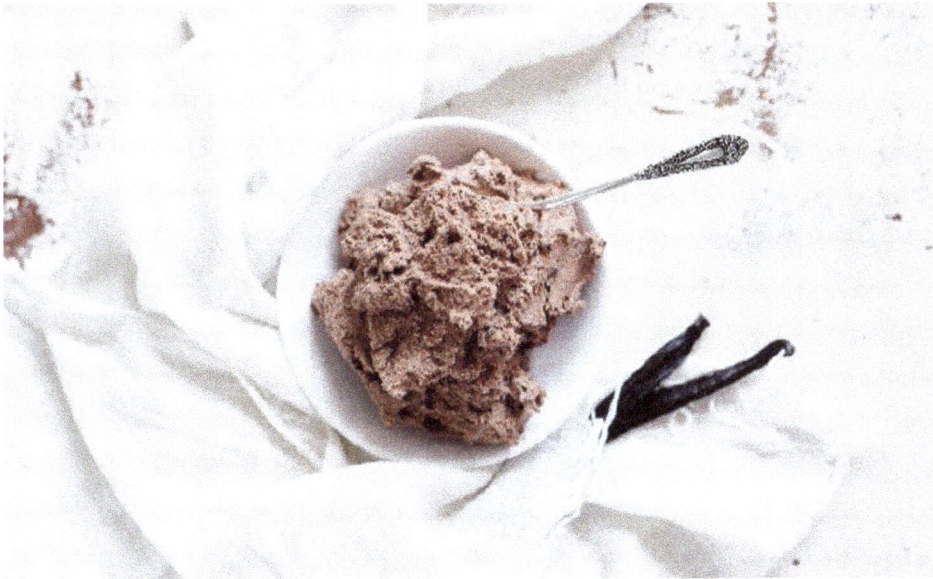

What's inside

- ½ avocado
- 1 banana
- 2 Tbs cacao powder
- 1 tsp vanilla

How to

1. Add all the ingredients to your food processor and blend until well combined.
2. Transfer into a container and chill in the fridge for about 15-30 minutes or until dessert time. Enjoy.

Variations

- For a minty After Eight style mousse, add 1 drop high quality peppermint essential oil.
- For a Jaffa chocolate mousse, add 1 drop high quality wild orange essential oil.

Straw-Yo Pralines

🕐 10 mins ⏳ 2 hrs 🍴 6 small pralines

This is my take on the German chocolate bar yogurette. Which is basically strawberry yogurt wrapped in chocolate. So easy yet sooooo good.

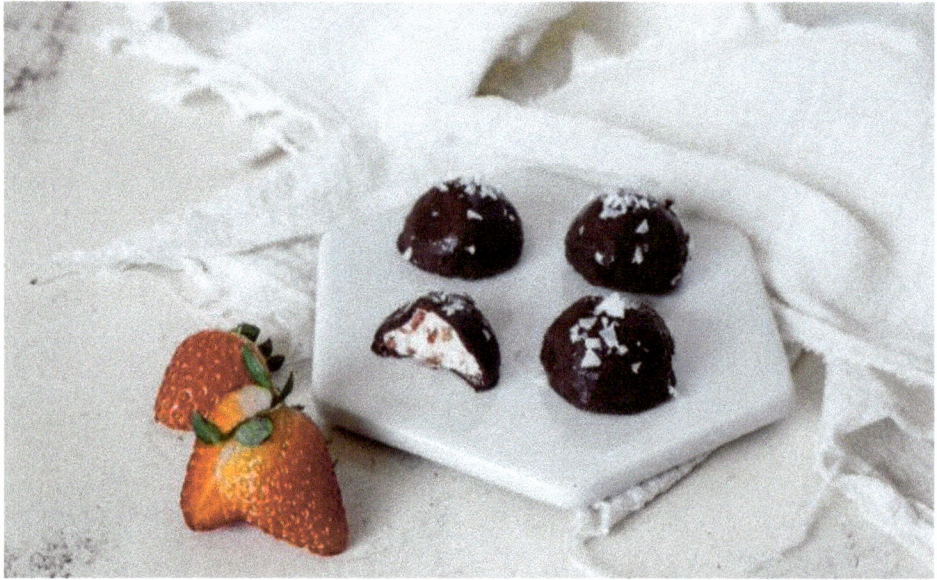

What's inside
- 2 Tbs coconut yogurt
- 2 Tbs freeze-dried strawberries
- 50g dairy-free dark chocolate

How to
1. With a spoon, fold the strawberries into the yogurt.
2. Pour the yogurt in an ice cube tray and freeze for 1-2 hours.
3. Once the yogurt is frozen, melt the chocolate and carefully coat the yogurt pralines in chocolate using two forks. Depending on your room temperature, you might have to do this in batches or keep the pralines on an ice pack to avoid them getting soft.
4. Once everything is covered, enjoy straight away or put them back into the freezer until it's dessert time.

Kitchen hack
- You can use fresh strawberries as well, it just turns out a little bit more watery.

Swap
- For an oil-free version: Swap the coconut yogurt for soy or nut-based yogurt.

Matcha Pralines

🕐 10 mins ⧗ 2 hrs 🍴 6 small pralines

Matcha, the Japanese ceremonial powdered green tea, reminds me of 2014, when hubby and I went on a spontaneous 4-day Japan trip for our first anniversary. It was amazing. If you ever get the chance—GO. My highlights – meditating on a little green island in the middle of Tokyo, the Golden Temple of Kyoto and the deers in Nara.

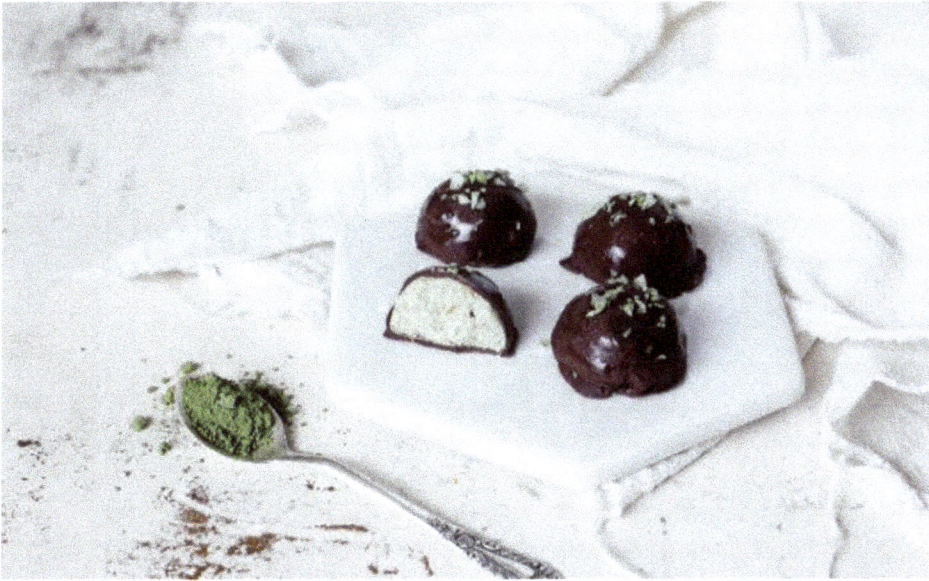

What's inside
- 2 Tbs coconut yogurt
- 1tsp matcha powder
- 50g dairy-free dark chocolate

How to
1. With a spoon, mix the yogurt and matcha powder until well combined.
2. Pour the yogurt into an ice cube tray and freeze for 1-2 hours.
3. Once the yogurt is frozen, melt the chocolate and carefully coat the yogurt pralines in chocolate using two forks. Depending on your room temperature, you might have to do this in batches or keep the pralines on an ice pack to avoid them getting soft.
4. Once everything is covered, enjoy straight away or put them back in the freezer until it's dessert time.

Swap
- For an oil-free version: Swap the coconut yogurt for soy or nut-based yogurt.

Choc-Yo Pralines

🕐 10 mins ⏳ 2 hrs 🍴 6 small pralines

Being married to a chocolate addict, I also had to create a double choc praline – he loves it.

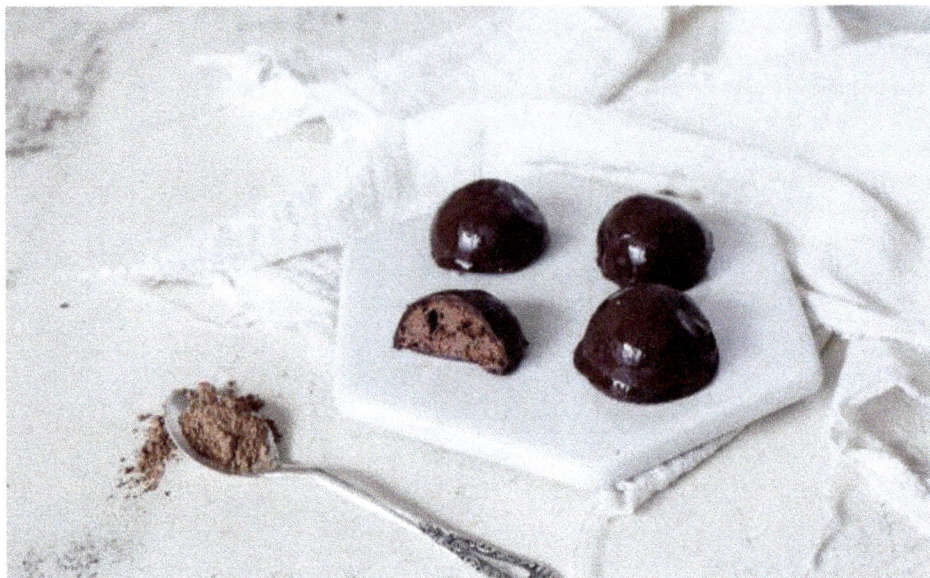

What's inside
- 2 Tbs coconut yogurt
- 1 tsp cacao powder
- 50g dairy-free dark chocolate

How to
1. With a spoon, mix the yogurt and cacao powder until well combined.
2. Pour the yogurt in an ice cube tray and freeze for 1-2 hours.
3. Once the yogurt is frozen, melt the chocolate and carefully coat the yogurt pralines in chocolate using two forks. Depending on your room temperature, you might have to do this in batches or keep the pralines on an ice pack to avoid them getting soft.
4. Once everything is covered, enjoy straight away or put them back into the freezer until it's dessert time.

Swap
- For an oil-free version: Swap the coconut yogurt for soy or nut-based yogurt.

NICE CREAM & SMOOTHIES

Banana Nice Cream

🕐 5 mins   ⧗ 0 mins   🍴 2

If I had known how easy self-made 100% sugar-free ice cream is, I would've started making it way before I went dairy-free. This Nice Cream is the perfect base to let out your kitchen creativity and start experimenting.

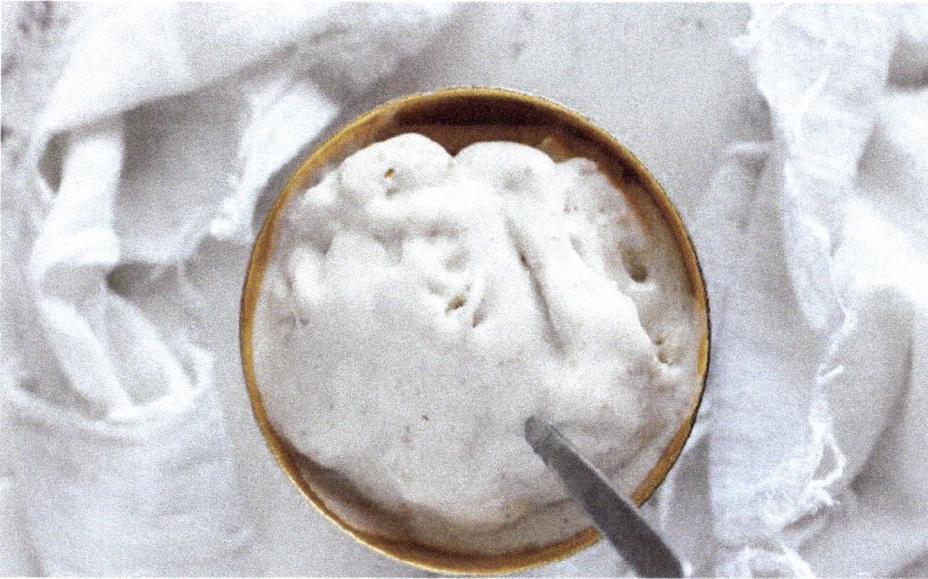

What's inside

- ¼ cup of your favourite mylk or water
- 3 frozen bananas, cut into pieces
- 2 Tbs peanut butter

How to

1. Blend all ingredients.
2. Occasionally turn the blender off and scrape down the fruit until you get a smooth texture. This might take about 2 minutes (depending on your blender).
3. Enjoy!

Kitchen hack

- Be careful not to blend for too long as the ice will turn into a sauce. If this happens, simply pour into a container and put in the freezer for 15 minutes.

Green Machine

🕐 5 mins   ⏳ 0 mins   🍴 2

I honestly believe every smoothie tastes better if you add some greens. This one is a tropical version for a lovely sunny summer day. Oh yum, spinach & pineapple go just soooo well together. #nom

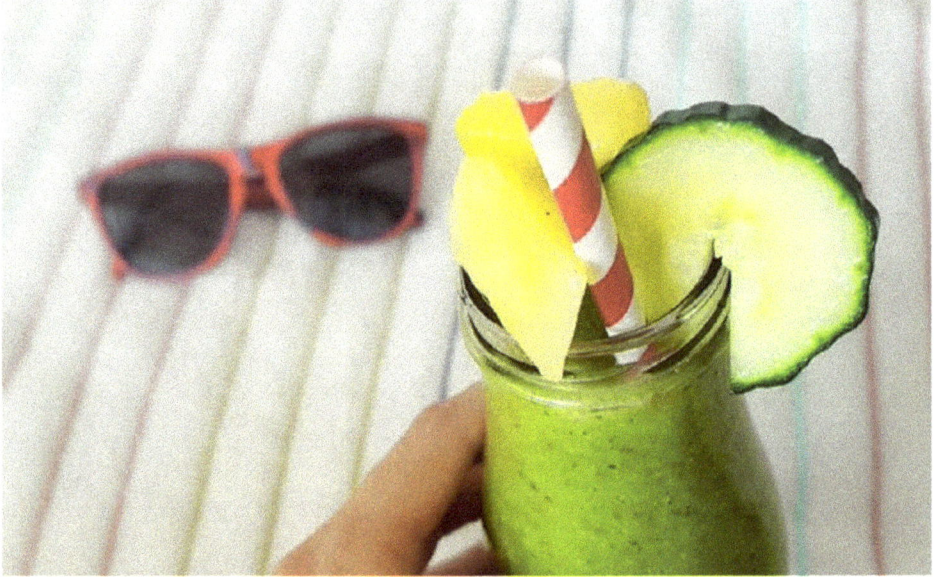

What's inside

- 1 cup almond mylk
- 1 cup spinach
- 1 avocado
- ½ cup frozen pineapple
- 1 cucumber
- 2 Tbs chia seeds

How to

1. Add everything to your blender, liquids first.
2. Blend until smooth.

Swap

- You can replace the almond mylk with water or your favourite mylk.

Green Salted Caramel

🕐 5 mins   ⧗ 0 mins   🍽 2 cups

As a peanut butter addict and leafy green junky, this is my absolute favourite smoothie. It has converted quite a few people to peanut butter by now. You definitely have to give it a try.

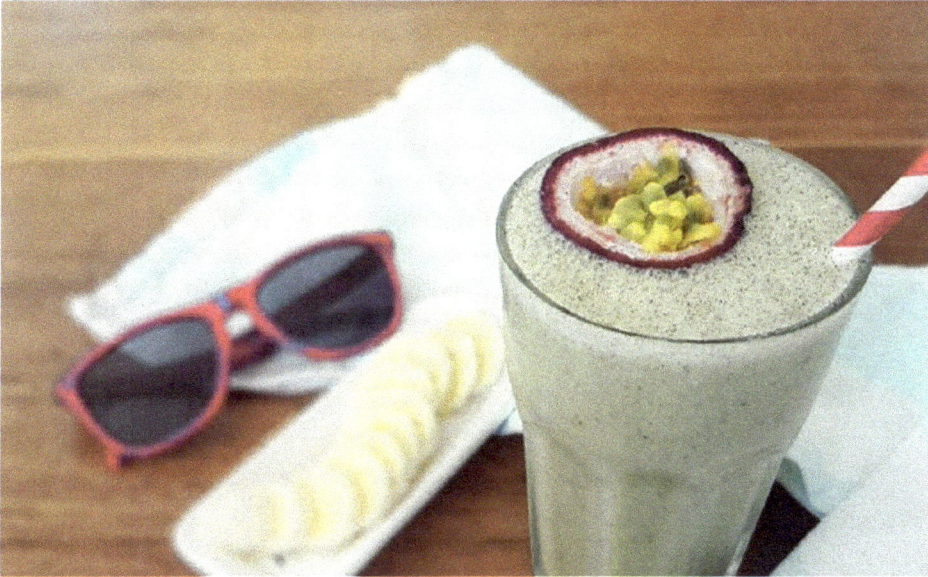

What's inside

- 1 cup water
- 1 small frozen banana (½ cup)
- ½ Lebanese cucumber (½ cup)
- 1 date
- 1 cup kale
- 3 Tbs peanut butter
- ½ tsp salt

How to

1. Add everything to your blender, liquids first.
2. Blend until smooth.

Kitchen hack

- To fill you up for a bit longer, simply add 1-2 tablespoons of flaxseeds - they'll do the trick.

Green Mango Lassi

🕐 5 mins　　⏳ 0 mins　　🍴 2

Have you ever ordered a mango lassi when you've been eating out at an Indian restaurant? How good is it? This combination of yogurt, mango and mint is all blended up to a cocktail-like green goddess – too good!

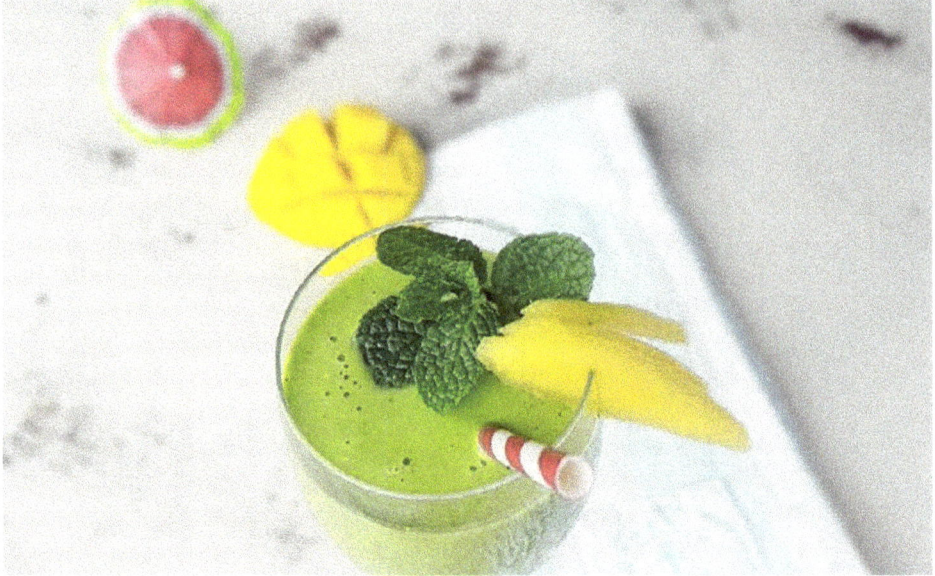

What's inside

- 1 cup rice mylk
- 1/3 cup coconut yogurt
- 1 frozen mango
- 1 cup spinach
- 3 mint springs

How to

1. Add everything to your blender, liquids first.
2. Blend until smooth.

Swap

- You can replace the rice mylk with water or your favourite mylk.

Rich Chocolate Smoothie

🕐 5 mins   ⧗ 0 mins   🍴 2

Beetroot and cacao – match made in heaven! Beautifully rich and flavoursome. Have you ever used the beetroot leaves? They are not just pretty, they are also super delicious and nourishing, plus using them in your smoothie will help to reduce food waste.

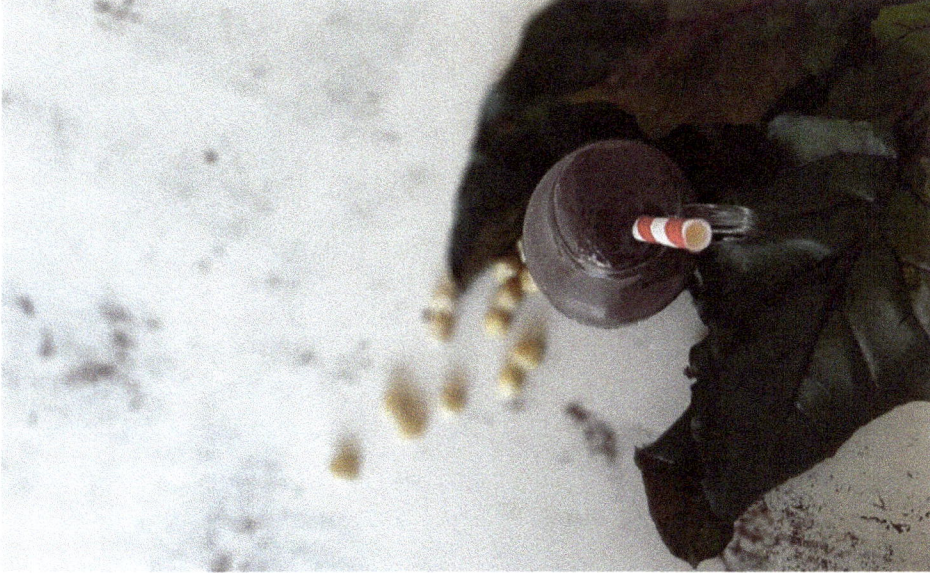

What's inside

- 1 cup rice mylk
- 1 cup beetroot leaves
- 1 zucchini
- 2 Tbs flaxseeds

- 2 Tbs cacao powder
- ¼ cup hazelnuts
- 2 frozen bananas
- 1 cup frozen berries

How to

1. Add everything to your blender, liquids first.
2. Blend until smooth.

Swap

- You can replace the rice mylk with water or your favourite mylk.

CHEAT SHEETS

I have created these cheat sheets to support you during your transition. Many people like to cut them out and either put them in their purse for when they go shopping, or put them on the fridge to support them daily as they cook. If you are reading this on your mobile device, you can simply screenshot the pages you like so you have them handy whenever you need them.

Cheat Sheets

My favourite replacements 135

Names of dairy 135

Swap guide 136

Shopping guide 136

Dairy-free staples 137

Meal Inspiration 137

Pantry Newbies 138

Pantry Keepers 138

Pantry Nasties 139

Nutritional information 141

Going out 141

Time & cost saving hacks 142

Dinner party ideas 143

Entertainer's guide 143

My fav replacements

Category	DIY	Brand
Milk (coffee)		
Milk (cereals)		
Yoghurt		
Butter		
Cooking cream		
Whipped cream		
Cheese (for eating raw)		
Cheese (for melting)		
Ice cream		
Chocolate		

i quit DAIRY

Names of dairy

Definitely milk containing

Butter butter - fat, oil, milk, solids

Casein casenate (like calcium, iron, magnesium or sodium casenate)

Cheese incl. cottage cheese and all animal-based cheeses, like goat/sheep

Cream incl. sour or whipped cream

Curds

Custard

Galactose

Ghee

Hydrolysates, Half & Half

Milk: incl. acidophilus, condensed, dry, evaporated, malted, sour, fat or non-fat milk, milk derivates, protein, powder or solids

Lact... lactalbumin, lactate solids, lactyc yeast, lactitol monohydrate, lactoferrin, lactoglobulin, lactose, lactulose

Nougat

Nisin preparation

Paneer

Recaldent

Rennet

Yogurt

Whey & Whey Protein (also galactose)

Potentially milk containing

Flavouring (artificial or natural), **Galactose, Lactic acid, Margarine, Pre- and probiotics, Protein**

i quit DAIRY

Swap guide

Old	New
Milk	Nut, soy, coconut, seed, grain or oat mylk or water
Butter milk	1-2 cups mylk + 1 Tablespoon apple cider vinegar or lemon juice
Yogurt	Coconut yoghurt & kefir, almond or soy yogurt, silken tofu or puddings made with chia, tapioca or sago pearls
Cheese	Nut or soy cheeses, nut butters or veggies like a thick slice of eggplant on pizza or avocado with nachos
Whipped cream	Coconut cream or yogurt, silken tofu, nut butter
Cooking cream	DIY (1:1 cashew-water mix), coconut cream, nut butter, tahini, silken tofu or flour-water mix
Sour cream	Dairy-free yogurt or self-made
Butter	Avocado, tahini, oils (olive, macadamia, coconut), even banana in baking
Ice cream	Sorbet, self-made nice cream, frozen fruit
Chocolate	Vegan chocolates or dark chocolates

Shopping guide

Category	Brands
Mylk	Bonsoy, Pure Harvest, Inside out, Nutty Bruce
Yogurt	Coyo, Nudie, Bondi
Snack	Chia Co (chia pods)
Cheese	Sprout & Kernel, Nozzarella (melting), Damona (feta and pepperjack), The Vegan Dairy, Botanical Cuisine
Spreads	Botanical Cuisine, Peace and Vegetables, Kehoe's
Nut butters	Food to Nourish, Mayvers, Loving Earth, Macro
Dips	Syndian, Organic Indulgence, Pilpel, Mama's
Chocolate	Pana Organic, Loving Earth, The Chocolate Yogi
Ice Cream	Coyo, Lux, Pana Organic, Over the Moo, Zebra
Protein Powders	Prana, Amazonia

Dairy-free staples

Food	Ingredients
Mylk	1 cup nuts + 4 cups water
Buttermilk	1 cup mylk + 1 Tbs lemon juice or apple cider vinegar
Cooking cream	1 cup nuts + 1 cup water
Sour Cream	2 cup nuts + 1 cup water + 5 Tbs lemon juice or apple cider vinegar
Cream cheese	1 cup nuts + ¼ cup water + nutritional yeast
Best nuts	Cashew nuts or almonds (soaked for 4-8 hours)

i quit .. **DAIRY**

Meal inspiration

Meal	Inspiration
Breakfast	• Overnight oats, cereals and porridge • Smoothie or smoothie bowls (açai bowls) • Fruit salad • Pancakes • Beans & Avocado on toast
Lunch	• Salad • Left-overs • Wraps • Sandwiches • Soups
Snack	• Fruit & nuts • Veggies with dip • Bliss balls • Falafel & hummus • Baked sweet potatoes
Dinner	• Curry • Stir-fry • Chili • BBQ & salad • Pasta
Dessert	• Nice cream • Dairy-free chocolate • Banana with peanut butter • Yoghurt or chocolate dipped frozen fruit • Mousse au chocolate

i quit .. **DAIRY**

Newbies (dairy-free pantry list)

Category	Foods
Nuts	Almond, brazil, cashew, macadamia, pecan, walnut
Seeds	Chia, flaxseeds, pumpkin (pepitas), sunflower, sesame
Soy	Organic & non GMO firm, silken & smoked tofu, tempeh & edamame beans
Staples	Nutritional yeast (aka nooch), vinegars (apple cider vinegar), tahini (sesame seed butter), nut butters (almond, cashew, peanut), tamari (or soy sauce), miso paste & coconut cream
Herbs & spices	Italian (oregano, basil, thyme), curry spice mix (good quality), paprika, turmeric, pepper, salt, cinnamon, cacao & vanilla powder
Fats	Avocados, nuts, nut oils, extra virgin coconut or olive oil
Sweetener	Dates, banana, coconut nectar or sugar, maple, agave or rice malt syrup

www.iqsdairy.com

Keepers (traditionally dairy-free)

Category	Foods
Wholefoods	Foods without a list of ingredients like veggies, fruits
Condiments	Ajvar, hummus, guacamole, salsa, jam, nut butters, mustard, tahini
Sauces	Worchester sauce, BBQ sauces, tomato sauces, chilli sauce, soy / tamari sauce
Dressings	Balsamic, French and Italian vinaigrette
Breakfast	Wholemeal, sourdough, pita bread, bagels, toasts, oats, cornflakes, vegemite, jams, Weet-Bix
Snacks	Veggies with dip, fruits, falafel, classic nachos & potato chips, wedges, olives, popcorn, rice cakes
Sweets	Dark chocolate, raw cakes, bliss balls, brownies & muffins (if traditionally baked with oil), sorbets, fruit ice, cocowhip
Drinks	Water, tea, juice, coffee (black), alcohol (incl beer, cider, spirits)

www.iqsdairy.com

Nasties (dairy foods 1/4)

The obvious

Milk	plain, skim, low-fat, flavoured, powdered, butter milk, condensed, evaporated, lactose free, infant formula, milk from cow, goat, sheep, camel, A2
Butter	
Chocolate	milk, flavoured, white, some dark
Cheese	hard, soft, ricotta, mozzarella, bocconcini, parmesan, mascarpone, cream cheese
Cream	whipped, thickened, cooking, sour cream, creme fraiche, ice cream
Quark	
Yogurt	

Nasties (dairy foods 2/4)

At second sight

Baked goods	Cupcakes, pastry (incl. pies, croissants) banana bread, brioches, wraps, cakes, pancakes
Bread spreads	Nutella, incl. some nut spreads
Soups	esp. creamed soups
Sweet snacks / breakfast	Muesli bars, chocolate bars, oat drinks, caramel, custard
Savoury snacks	Flavoured chips and nachos, popcorn, garlic bread
Dips & Sauces	Tzatziki, low fat versions of aioli or guacamole
Curries	Might contain ghee, butter or cream
Protein powders	often whey based
Roasted veggies or sizzling mushrooms	Glazed with butter
Pasta sauces	Alfredo, carbonara, pesto, mac n cheese
Salad dressings	Caesar, ranch, yogurt

Nasties (dairy foods 3/4)

The not so obvious (brand dependent)

Processed meats	Marinades, cold cuts, salami, sticks and sausages
Processed meals	esp. frozen pasta, rice dishes or soups
Tomato sauces	Restaurants sometimes add butter (double check)
Fries	Sometimes contain milk powder
Potato mash	Butter and milk are common ingredients
Dips & sauces	Hummus, guacamole, gravy
Gluten-free products	
Dark Chocolates	Cadbury and others
Coconut products	Some dairy products are coconut flavoured like coconut milk powder, condensed milk or yogurt
Medications	esp. in tablets and probiotics
Soy products	Like some cheeses and soy chai latte powders

i quit **DAIRY**

Nasties (dairy foods 4/4)

The hidden ones (esp relevant if allergic)

Dairy-free products	Due to cross contamination
Dairy-free yogurts	In the cultures
Probiotics	Look for vegan options
Flavourings	Natural & artificial
Wine	Some brands use milk in the fining process

i quit **DAIRY**

Nutritional information

Category	Foods
Calcium	Leafy greens (esp kale, broc choy & broccoli), soy beans, tahini, almonds Absorption booster: Always have calcium rich foods together with some vitamin C, like lemon, orange or capsicum.
Potassium	Sweet potatoes, bananas, coconut water, avocados & spinach
Vitamin D	Sunshine is by far the best source of Vitamin D, better than any other food source. Make sure you expose your skin (no sunscreen) for at least 15min every day and take a supplement in winter
Magnesium	Spinach, chards, pumpkin seeds, dark chocolate, Epsom salt baths
Probiotics	Fermented vegetables, like kombucha, raw sauerkraut, probiotic powders

Going out

Category	Foods
Vegan, Raw	100 % dairy-free. Enjoy anything off the menu
Paleo	95% dairy-free, watch out for butter, yogurt and parmesan.
Organic & wholefoods	Meals cooked from scratch. Usually happy make changes to meet your requirements.
Asian (Chinese, Malaysian, Thai)	Traditionally dairy-free. Coconut milk instead of dairy products
Lebanese	Mostly dairy-free, watch out for labna and some yogurt dips
Indian	Mostly okay, just check if they use yogurt or ghee in their curries
Italian	Pizza without cheese (some offer vegan cheese or sliced eggplant instead), Pasta with tomato sauce - double check that they use olive oil not butter
Note	Always check with the chef, the waiters might not be aware about your specific needs and the recipe. Some restaurants cook with butter or add some dairy to the salad dressing etc.

Time saving hacks

Wholefoods faster than restaurant or take-home

Preparation
- Soak rice for dinner in the morning (cuts cooking time in half)
- Overnight oats with fresh fruit (energising grab and go in the morning)

Get a food processor
And your veggies will be cut in a blink

15-20 min recipe repertoire
Don't cook for hours – get quick, easy & yummy recipes

Plan ahead
Meal plan = no worries, no extra shopping = more time

Batches
Cook in batches, freeze leftovers for those busy days
Cut veggies in batches for salad, wraps / sandwiches

Cost saving hacks

Hack	Details
DIY	• Mylks • Cooking cream • Dips • Nut butters (only if high-speed blender)

Cooking	• Use the whole thing
	  - Celery leaves in salad or as spice
	  - Cauliflower stalk in potato mash
	  - Broccoli stalk in stir-fry
	• Cook in batches & freeze
	• Fry with water not expensive oils
	• Buy coconut cream not milk (if same price) add ½ cup water = coconut milk

Shopping	• Join a co-op • Local Farmer markets • Buy with the seasons • Buy in bulk (esp. nuts & seeds) • Buy organic berries frozen • Get the ugly bunch • 2nd choice fruit & veg – it's all just food
Freezing	• Bananas • Avocados • Leftovers (even wine) • Double use your beautiful herbal teas

Dinner party ideas

Cuisine	Course	Meal
Italian	Starter	Bruschetta & olives
	Main	Pasta bolognese with side salad
	Dessert	Newtella banana pizza
Mexican	Starter	Nacho with guacamole
	Main	Chilli with dairy-free queso
	Dessert	Chilli chocolate
Indian	Starter	Papadam with dip
	Main	Curry
	Dessert	Sticky rice with mango
America	Starter	Mac n cheese
	Main	Burger
	Dessert	Banana peanut butter nice cream
Summer / Picnic	Starter	Quinoa salad
	Main	Zoodles with raw capsicum sauce
	Dessert	Smoothie

Entertainer's guide

Course	Meal
Starter	1 Rainbow salad with vegan cheese board
	2 Soup
	3 Rice paper rolls
	4 Mezze platter
	Dolmades, falafel, carrots, cucumbers, roasted capsicum, olives and hummus
	5 Antipast with ciabatta and olive oil
	Olives, roasted eggplant and capsicum
Main	1 Curry or Stir-fry
	2 Filling salads
	3 BBQ or oven veggies with dips
	4 Pasta or Pizzas
	5 Chilli
Dessert	1 Fruit salad
	2 Chia pudding
	3 Chocolate dipped fruits
	4 Nice cream
	5 Raw cake

i quit DAIRY

RECIPE FRAMEWORKS

Sometimes all we need are rough guidelines. These frameworks are here for you to spark your own creativity, allow you to play around and create YOUR favourite recipes. Explore some of the ingredients, start playing around, fail, try again until you are equipped with your own dairy-free recipes. Creating meals, is meant to be fun and playful, that's how we infuse our food with love and joy, that's when it tastes amazing.

Recipe Framewoks

Mylk 145

Nice Cream 145

Smoothie 146

Dressing 146

Spread 147

Chocolate 147

Mylk

Liquid (2 cups)	Base (¼ - ½ cup)	Flavour (1 - 3 teaspoons)	Sweetener (optional)
Water	**Nuts** (soaked) almonds, cashew, brazil, macadamia	Vanilla	Banana
Coconut water	**Seeds** sunflower, pepitas, hemp	Cacao	Date
	Grains rice, quinoa, buckwheat	Cinnamon	Grapes
	Coconut fresh or dried	Turmeric	
		Citrus zest	
		Ginger	

i quit DAIRY

Nice Cream

Frozen Base (1 cup)	Liquid (¼ cup)	Extra kick (optional)	Toppings (optional)
Banana (works best)	Coconut water	**Nut butter** Almond, peanut, cashew	Cacao nibs
Mango	Mylk	Cacao powder	Coconut flakes
Açai	**Yogurt** dairy-free of course	Coconut butter	**Fresh fruit** cherries, blue-, goji, rasp- & strawberries
Pineapple		Cookies	Nuts
Peach			Melted chocolate
Melon			Rose petals
Avocado + Zucchini for a low fructose version (Avocado is best to mix with lime)			

i quit DAIRY

Smoothie

Greens (1 cup)	Veg / Fruit* (1 - 1½ cups)	Liquid (½ - 1 cup)	Power (optional)
Kale	**Vegetables** avocado, beetroot, broccoli, carrot, celery, cucumber, zucchini	**Water**	**Seeds** chia, flax, hemp
Spinach		**Mylk**	**Nuts** almonds, brazil, cashew, peanut
Rocket	**Fruits** apple, banana, berries, kiwifruit, mango, papaya, pear, pineapple, watermelon	**Coconut water**	**Powders** açai, cacao, carob, cardamom, cinnamon, coffee, ginger, hemp, oats, maca, lucuma, psyllium husk, plant-based protein, turmeric
Cos		**Coconut milk**	
Mixed salad			
Herbs coriander, parsley, mint, dandelion			

*fresh or frozen

i quit DAIRY

www.iquitdairy.com

Dressing

Base (¼ cup)	Acidity (2 tablespoons)	Liquid (optional)	Flavour (optional)
Mustard	**Vinegar** apple cider, red wine, brown rice, white wine, sherry, cider	**Water**	**Berries**
Nut butter almond, cashew		**Mylk**	**Garlic & onion**
Miso	**Citrus juice** lemon, grapefruit, orange	**Olive oil**	**Herbs** basil, chilli, curry, oregano, parsley, pepper, rosemary, turmeric
Tahini			**Sweetener** agave syrup, berries, lime, balsamic vinegar, brown rice syrup, coconut nectar, stevia

i quit DAIRY

www.iquitdairy.com

Spreads

Base (1 cup)	Liquid (¼ cup)	Flavour (1–3 tablespoons)	Herbs (optional)
Nuts (soaked) almonds, cashew, hazelnut, macadamia	Water	Nutritional yeast	Basil
	Lemon juice	Garlic & onion	Chilli
	Coconut milk	Tomato (fresh, dried)	Dill
or		Paprika (fresh, powder)	Oregano
½ Tomato paste +		Curry	Parsley
½ Seeds (soaked) sunflower, pepitas		Cacao	Pepper
			Rosemary
			Thyme

i quit DAIRY

Chocolate

Base (½ cup)	Crunch (½ cup)	Cacao (¼ cup)	Sweetener (2-4 tablesp.)	Deco (optional)
Cacao butter	Nut butter almond, cashew, hazelnut	Cacao powder	Brown rice syrup	Cacao nibs
Coconut oil		Rice milk powder for white chocolate	Coconut nectar	Chilli flakes
	Coconut butter		Coconut sugar	Citrus zest
			Pure maple syrup	Coconut shreds
				Cornflakes
				Dried fruit
				Nuts
				Rose petals
				Salt flakes

i quit DAIRY

Thank You

There is only one person I would like to thank right now and that is YOU.

Thank you so much for listening to your body. Thank you for diving into your dairy-free journey. And thank you for supporting our mission to help people discover the joy of dairy-free living by reading this book. We hope the content helped you or a loved one.

Sometimes when I finish a book, I have a message for the author. I would like to share how the book helped me or I feel like I would like to give back. In either case, I'd love to hear from you. Please send me an email to kris@iquitdairy.com – with the subject "I read *I Quit Dairy*".

I created this project to build a community. My vision is that as our service helps people, some of those people will feel inspired to give back. They will share, they will inspire others, they will provide new recipes, they could create meet-ups, they may even become health-professionals or start their own businesses, create dairy-free products aka. expand the 2nd milk universe and partner with us.

Wherever your journey leads you. From deep down in my heart I wish you all the best for your health and your life. May it be filled with joy, freedom and gratitude. Thank you for crossing my path and getting a taste for the 2nd milk universe.

I am sending you a big wave of love, health and energy.

Sunny wishes,

Kris x

Find out more on *www.iquitdairy.com*

@iquitdairynow

KRIS GOETZ Once an accident survivor, unable to walk, Kris decided to take her life into her own hands. After trying many methods, she finally healed herself through a combination of dairy-free nutrition, meditation and mind-set work, and is now living the life of her dreams. Filled with energy and dedication she is on a mission to inspire others to follow her example.

Kris Goetz is now the CEO/founder of *I Quit Dairy,* an experienced mindset coach, author and TEDx speaker. During her 15 years of extensive research she has learnt from thought leaders such as Dr. Bernard, Dan Buettner and Louise Hay whose guidance helped to cure her chronic headaches, a major hip injury, reverse an auto-immune disease and lose 15kgs. If she is not speaking at health and wellness symposiums in Australia or Europe, working with her team on *I Quit Dairy*, you might find her surfing with her friends, meditating next to a tree or travelling the world with her soulmate, Markus.

Going dairy-free was a major change in her life. Now she wants to give back. Through *I Quit Dairy* she is helping others live a healthier lifestyle so that they too can ultimately achieve their goals in life.

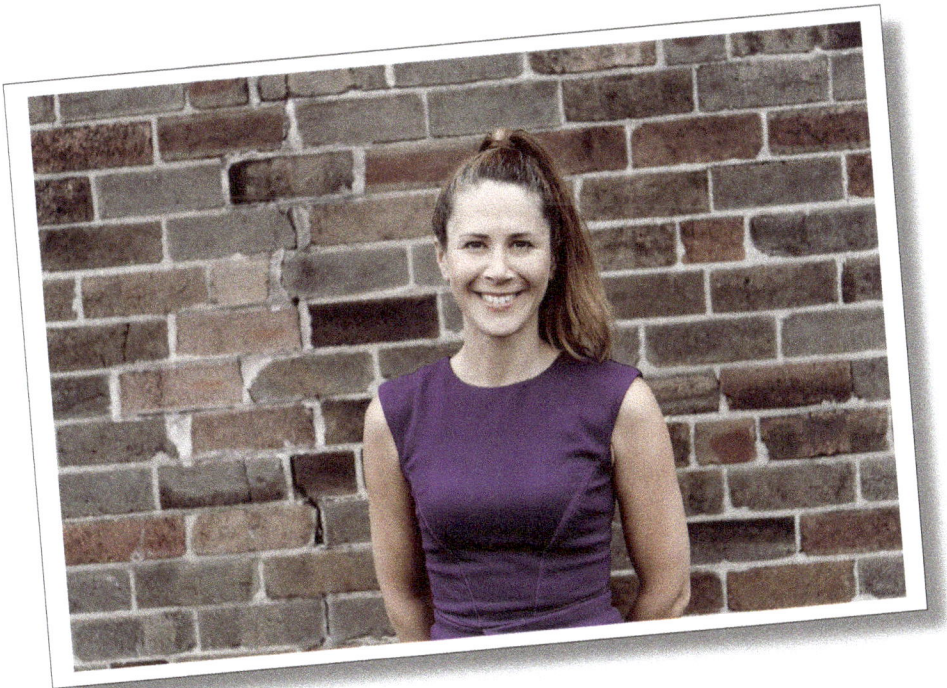

www.ingramcontent.com/pod-product-compliance
Lightning Source LLC
Chambersburg PA
CBHW051617030426
42334CB00030B/3228